Get Back in Shape After 50:

Jump Start the Second Half of Your Life

By

Richard Schuller

Library of Congress-in Publication Data has been applied for

Mid Life Hard Body book

Cover design by Rocking Book Covers

Photography by Ian Shadburne, Richard Schuller and Susan Shadburne

For additional free information, equipment sources and nutrition guidance go to

    www.MidLifeHardBody.com

Disclaimer

You should recognize that any exercise program involves some element of risk. You should consult with your physician or health care professional to see if this program is something you can do without endangering your health, and for diagnosis and treatment of illness, injuries and for advice regarding medications.

While exercise is normally beneficial, it is important that you undertake knowing that you do not have any health conditions that may be aggravated or damaged by activities in this program. The author and Mid Life Hard Body, LLC shall have neither liability nor responsibility to any person or entity with respect to any damage or injury alleged to be caused directly or indirectly by the information contained in this book.

You should never discontinue taking medications prescribed by your doctor without specific consultation with your doctor. You should obtain clearance from your doctor before you undertake any program of exercise as the activities may be too strenuous or dangerous for some people.

Before making any changes to your personal diet and nutrition habits it is recommended that you consult with your physician or health care professional. The nutrition information and suggestions in this book are for informational purposes only. While every attempt has been made to verify the accuracy of information provided in all portions of this book, neither the author, nor any affiliate s/partners assume any responsibility for errors, inaccuracies, or omissions.

The information contained in this book is not intended for the treatment or prevention of disease, nor as a substitute for medical treatment. The nutrition information in this book should not be adopted without consultation with a physician or your health care professional. Use of information contained in any portion of this book is the sole responsibility of the reader. Neither the author nor any affiliate s/partner is responsible or liable for any harm or injury resulting from the exercises, nutrition advice, or personal management strategies.

To Susan, the light of my world

Table of Contents

Introduction

Get back into shape over age 50

You are "over 50" and you feel your age. You want to look youthful and vibrant. You don't want to feel like your time is past. You know that you can be in a lot better physical condition.

Right now, you face a choice. You can start working to make major upgrades in your physical condition. Or, you can resign yourself to progressive decline and accept a greatly diminished quality of life as time goes by.

You have a choice.

You may have been in good physical condition before and want to get back that great "feel" of being strong and agile. But…you are over 50. You wonder "can I get back to looking and feeling great…or even close?"

Not only yes…but HELL YES!!!!

It is possible to:

- Look *sensational!!!*
- Feel like you are 20+ years younger
- Have seemingly endless energy
- Be amazingly strong
- Have outrageous physical vitality
- Keep all of this *indefinitely!!!*

Most people have the potential to get into spectacular physical condition after age 50. It is even possible to get in great condition at a much later age….I should know….I'm 78 as I write this and as you can see from my pictures, I'm in great condition…and I feel like I'm 35!

But, this is about you and what you want to accomplish.

Being fit is a major life destiny decision

If you are over 50 (or 60 or 70 or beyond), now is the time to get rolling on a fitness program that will change the rest of your life. **Choosing to be fit is a major life destiny decision.**

If you choose to build your strength and fitness as a 50+ year old, you have made a decision that will impact *how all the rest of your life unfolds*. When you are fit, there is an overwhelming probability that you will enjoy an outstanding quality of life for decades.

Not only do you enjoy the benefits years from now, you get an *immediate* impact on how you look and feel. Being fit will have a *huge positive impact* on your physical viability 2 months from now, 2 years from now, 10 years from now and even 25 years from now.

This is in direct contrast to people who will simply allow nature to take its course and gradually succumb to the ravages of age.

People who don't choose to be fit face bleak future of chronic illness, getting progressively feebler, gobbling medications, and living from one doctor visit to the next.

Most people take the easy path and ignore fitness training. One day they wake up and discover that they have gradually become a wreck. At that point they may try heroic measures to reverse their condition. But, to their everlasting chagrin their efforts are too little and way too late.

It would have been relatively easy and far less painful to have built a fit and resilient body years before. But, they couldn't be bothered back then. When they finally realize what they should have done, it is too late.

As I said, **choosing to be fit after age 50 is a major *life destiny* decision**.

In addition to keeping the ravages of aging at bay, being fit has a huge payoff for you *in the present*. You get to enjoy feeling and looking great NOW!

What does "great quality of life" mean to you?

Here are a few answers from people over 50 who I have coached:

- looking great
- Feeling physically strong
- Moving easily with balance, power, and grace
- Never having to think about chronic illness or limiting conditions
- Feeling good in your own skin
- Having fun doing physical activities
- Feeling physically confident
- not having any serious health issues
- having off the chart physical vitality.
- doing what you want without having to worry about physical limitations.
- having fun buying new clothes because you know they will look great on you

You probably have your own list, but I'm betting that some or all the answers listed above would be on it in one form or another.

The cool thing is that for the vast majority of people over age 50, these things *can* be achieved.

If you currently feel far away from enjoying this quality of life, the program in this book can get you on the road back to where you want to be.

Real fitness for 50+

I have found that most fitness programs designed for "people over 50" are pathetic. It seems that most are written by people in their 30's and 40's who appear to believe that anyone over 50 is both feeble and fragile.

The authors seem to assume you could never lift anything heavier than a roll of toilet paper. Heavy weights are to be avoided, and nothing more vigorous than "brisk walking" is advised for cardio activity.

Some of these programs for "adults" even go so far as to say that lots of exercise will "age you more rapidly" than if you sat on your butt. What utter rubbish!

As I write this, I'm 78 years old. I have been training hard for 60+ years. If any exercises were going to age me prematurely, I would have been in the ground a *long* time ago.

Instead, I have the body that is *decades* younger than my calendar age. I have NO chronic physical impairments or injuries. I don't take any prescription drugs. I'm strong to the point where I still compete in powerlifting, have the aerobic capacity of a hockey player and I have the energy of a 30-year-old.

This didn't happen by magic. I'm not some genetic freak. It DID happen through regular exercise, good nutrition, and proper mindset that I'll tell you about in this book.

In my view, the idea that people over age 50 are doomed to decline is total crap. I have trained a lot of men and women over age 50. I have seen that these folks can accomplish some extraordinary physical feats.

This program is for you IF....

You are a high achiever

- Designed for busy, high achieving people, who have crammed work schedules, families, and a social life.

- This program focuses on the "whole person": exercise, nutrition and mindset as opposed to exercise exclusively.
- Designed to be time efficient. Lots of return for every exercise performed.

You are focused on long term success

- Help you become progressively stronger and more athletic as you move through a sequence of courses.
- Wherever you start, this is designed to help you move up the chain from beginner to intermediate then advanced trainee and possibly even to elite performer.

You want "life skills" not just exercise

- Instead of a specific "diet" this program emphasizes changing major eating/nutrition habits.
- Designed to help you master the *life skill* of "being fit" that you will be able to use for decades.
- Will help expand your consciousness and enrich your life experience by helping you reconnect you to your physicality and what it "feels" like to be in great condition.

Proven to work for age 50+

- Designed and validated by the author who has been astonishingly fit for five decades even though he had a very demanding career as a scientist and executive, as well as a family and social life.
- Proven to work by the author and the regiments of people he has coached
- Uses measures of strength, body mass and athleticism to track progress rather than trivial measures such as "counting steps" or guessing at "calories burned".
- Based on long tested principles that work, not on the latest re-packaged fitness fad
- Cost effective by avoiding purchase of unnecessary or ineffective equipment.

Fitness is a life skill

Getting and *staying fit* and healthy is a *skill*. To become skilled, you must *learn what to do* and then *do it*. Skill is developed through hard work, study, and reflection. It does not just *happen* to you.

Learning by itself is not enough. Too many people appear to think that learning something is enough. It is learning and *applying what you learn* that brings results.

As you go through this program remember **you are the master of your own destiny.**

You have *chosen* to become strong and fit.

You are "the boss" of building your fitness skills so that you get progressively stronger and more fit.

You are *not* being *forced* to do some "boot camp" type workout run by a psychotic trainer who shrieks commands at you while you thrash around trying to rid yourself of ass fat.

You will *not* be "put on a diet" that prevents you from eating "things you want" and living in the private hell of constant self-denial.

You have the *power* and are *choosing* to *master the skills of how to transform and care for yourself.*

My job is to help you achieve what you want.

Thus, each month you will take on a slightly more demanding challenge. Your progress will come from building on the accumulated work you do.

At the end of three months, you will be amazed at the things you do easily that seemed impossible at the start. That is just the start of what you can accomplish.

Create your "vision"

You need to create a clear vision of what you intend to accomplish and a clear picture of who you will become.

Positive change happens when you focus on *what you want!*

Your vision becomes the reason you will work hard. It is your "because".

You should be as specific as possible. Define what your life will be like, how you will feel, what you want to become 24/7/365. This should include your appearance, vigor, energy, strength, mental focus, and so forth.

A clear vision of what you are building toward will be critical in the coming months. It will sustain you in difficult times and keep you on course. It will keep you out of the vagueness and "fog" of moving toward an unclear objective.

You should remember that your being fit and healthy is not just about the benefits you get.

Your being in top shape is *extremely* important to everyone who loves you and counts on you. When you are strong and healthy you will be "on deck" for your family, friends, co-workers, or others close to you.

Being in great condition means that you dramatically reduce the chances that your family (or someone else) will have to care for you as you age.

Being fit is also patriotic. How can that be? It means that you as a fit and healthy person put far less demand on the health care system. You *contribute* to society instead of sucking off resources to treat preventable ailments.

Organization of the course

The reconditioning program here is divided into three one-month segments.

Each month you will get new instruction in three areas:

- Exercise
- Nutrition
- Motivation and Mindset

Each of these factors play a critical role in your success. They are interrelated, and it is impossible to succeed without working on all three.

Each month you develop certain skills. The month following, you add to your skill set. In this way after three months you have made major changes to your body, you're eating patterns and how you think about the process getting and staying fit.

Here is a quick overview of the program.

Physical training

This program involves both weight training and aerobics training. This is to build a body that has both physical strength and cardiovascular fitness.

Every month you will get a new training program for both weights and cardio.

Weight training is essential to build healthy muscle tissue. Being physically strong is essential to fully enjoy every day life. You can "do things" without having to think about whether you are strong enough.

If you want to look good, weight training is essential to build an attractive physique.

The health benefits of weight training are enormous. For starters healthy muscle tissue can prevent degenerative medical conditions such as Type II diabetes, hypertension, elevated cholesterol, and heart disease.

Weight training is also essential to build strong bones and connective tissue. Weightlifting can actually reverse (or prevent) osteoporosis.

Aerobic training has dramatic positive impacts on both appearance and serious health issues.

Aerobics can have a massive impact on health of the heart, lungs, and circulatory system. A huge body of research over the past half century has established that aerobic training will reduce the risk of heart attacks and stroke. Recent research has established aerobic training as critical in preventing dementia.

Aerobic training contributes to developing an athletic looking physique. Because the entire body is involved in aerobic movements, one of the results is an overall fit appearance.

Nutrition

The nutrition program in this course is designed to help you develop the *habit patterns* that will allow you to have the best nutrition for you without constant stressing or decision making.

This comes down to dialing in some simple rules that you follow day after day.

Each month I'll provide some simplified guidance on basic approaches you can use to have a healthy eating program that will help you lose fat (if needed) and build your overall fitness.

I don't give you a "diet" for a couple reasons.

First, being on a diet is like holding your breath. You can force yourself to do it for a while, but eventually you must gasp for breath. Dieting is a lot like this. Discipline will keep you on it, until it won't.

Second, diets often feel like they are being "imposed" on you by some outside force bent on denying you from having the foods you crave the most. This means that proper eating is done because some "authority" is forcing you to comply with "the rules"

It is no wonder that after a few months, most people on a diet revert to their old eating patterns. Very often they and put all the fat they lost and a bunch more.

This program is based on the notion that you will embrace good eating patterns because it is part of what you have chosen to do as a fit person. Eating properly is your choice, not something dictated by an evil witch from The Diet Planet.

If you develop good habits you will routinely "do the right thing" without thinking.

Mindset

Each month I'll show you how you can use your mind to harness forces that will power your quest for being fit, strong and healthy. Mobilizing the power of your mind and spirit will make you unstoppable.

Changing patterns that have been "comfortable" or "regular" produces a lot of stress and blowback. You have established a life pattern that is "normal" for you.

Your body expects to be fed in a certain way, your friends expect you to follow a certain eating/socializing pattern and your family is used to you "the way you are".

When you make big changes in any area, expect blowback from many sources.

Mobilizing the power of your mind begins with daily commitment.

You are establishing a "new normal".

Each day you must look in the mirror and re-motivate yourself to get stronger, fitter, better looking and more committed. One of my favorite quotes sums it up:

> "People often say that motivation doesn't last. Well, neither does bathing. That's why we recommend it daily." - Zig Zigler

The most important single thing you can do to succeed is be *persistent*. Keeping at your task regardless of the headwinds will bring you success.

Making lasting changes requires not only motivation, but focused mental effort. You must believe you can make the changes you want and overcome thought patterns that tell you that change is impossible.

This is where the "growth mentality" comes in. Many people have their best intentions crippled by a mindset that tells them they cannot achieve what they want because of their own inherent limitations. This is the fixed mindset.

The growth mindset has been clearly documented by research over the past two decades. It establishes that there is *no way to know beforehand what you can accomplish if you work at it.*

Before you Start Working Out

It is important that you be examined by a doctor to ensure that you are healthy enough to do an exercise program. At age 50+ you may have some conditions that need to be addressed before it is safe for you to begin working out.

This is particularly true if you have suffered a heart attack or stroke.

If you have some chronic injuries, such as knee problems, shoulder problems, back issues, etc. you should be worked on by a physical therapist so that you will have no limitations on the exercise movements you can do.

If you are diabetic, hypoglycemic or have thyroid problems, you must to get a doctor's guidance on how to do the exercise program.

Training Issues

You need to determine where you will do your workouts. Some prefer the flexibility of training at a gym, while others prefer to train at home. Each has certain advantages. See Appendix A for guidance on setting up a home gym.

If you are considering joining a gym, I have also included a section on how to select a gym that will work best for you. (Appendix D)

I have also included a chapter on training with bodyweight only. As most of you know, it is possible to get a great workout without any equipment. Bodyweight training is a great complement to regular weight training. It is also handy to use if you are traveling and don't have access to your regular equipment. See Appendix E.

You are also likely to have your regular routine interrupted by travel for vacation or business. See Appendix B for advice on how to train while traveling.

Then there are the minor aches and pains you get from training. See Appendix C for a quick primer on treating routine minor injuries you get while training.

Who is offering all this advice?

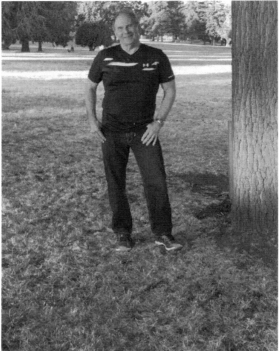

Oh…this is me…the 78-year-old who is handing out advice on how to be fit over age 50. I have 28 years' experience in being "over 50", and 63 years of physical fitness training. Started lifting weights in 1955 (gasp!). Played eight different sports. Competed in powerlifting from age 48 to 73…and going back to it. Competitive runner age 25 to age 47…still run some. Played all the "ball sports" as a kid and into middle age. Had a lot of fun. Feel like I'm a fit and healthy 35 year old…well….maybe 40.

My professional career was as a scientist, manager and executive in a private research and development company. I had to do a LOT of travel, both national and international. I also had a packed personal and family life. I was, and still am, a "high achiever".

Being extremely fit enabled me to be both more productive at work and more present and involved with my family. Training helped keep me grounded and helped my mind "get in the flow".

A Dozen Frequently Asked Questions (FAQ's)

If you are just beginning your quest to get in good condition, you will probably have some questions about what you should be doing. Here are a few FAQ's that may be on your mind.

1. **Are you ever too old to start physical training?** No! There are many examples of people in their mid-90's starting physical fitness programs and building both strength and endurance. Almost everyone who starts training in their 50's can benefit greatly. Incredible success is *possible*. However, consistent hard work is *necessary*.

2. **Is weight training necessary to get into good condition?** The simple answer is "yes". Some form of *resistance training* is necessary for someone to get in good condition. Weight training is the simplest to use when getting started and gives the biggest return on your investment of time and effort.

3. **There are many different workout routines, which is best?** There is no such thing as a "perfect" workout routine. When I was competing in powerlifting we used to joke that the "best" workout was the one you were not doing. There are a lot of different weight training workouts. Some are good for beginners and others only appropriate for advanced lifters. All of them require mastering the fundamental moves that are included in this book. Do the programs in this book, and you will get good results.

4. **Can getting in shape reverse the aging process?** Getting in good physical condition can significantly slow how rapidly you "age". One huge impact is slowing or reversing chronic degenerative conditions such as diabetes, heart disease, obesity, osteoporosis, circulatory problems, muscle degeneration, and arthritis. A fit lifestyle can produce a body (and mind) that are decades younger than your calendar age.

5. **Which diet is the best for losing fat and getting in shape?** There is no "perfect" diet for everyone. There are many different diet plans that can lead to success. Each person is a little different, and they will respond to alternative nutrition approaches differently. The most accurate answer to this question is that the "best" diet for you is the one you will *actually use*. It doesn't do you any good to "know" about a diet plan, but not practice it.

6. **How can I avoid getting hurt while getting back in shape?** This is an important issue that is often ignored. The best way to limit your chances for injury is to begin doing training that is within your capability but doesn't require you to do things your body can't handle. Training routines such as the ones in this book focus on doing training that can be both challenging and safe at the same time. It is harmful for a beginning trainee to try to do something that is far beyond

their capability. Over time, spectacular progress is possible. However, it is important to begin doing workouts that are well within your capability.

7. **Do I need to join a gym?** The simple answer is that you can set do your training at home, at a friend's house, at a company workout facility, in a gym, or anywhere you can have access to the equipment you need. The main benefit of a gym is having a big selection of equipment without having to buy the gear yourself. Home gym's offer the convenience of being able to train without traveling somewhere. The main drawback is usually that there is a limited amount of equipment. Buying equipment for a home gym can be expensive and a poor investment if you don't get the right stuff. (See Appendix A).

8. **Do I need a personal trainer?** If you follow the instructions in this book, you do not need a personal trainer. You can master the foundations of fitness training on your own by carefully following the lessons included here. Most people start working out without having a personal trainer.

9. **Is aerobic training necessary if I lift weights?** A resounding "yes". There are two critical components to being fit over age 50. One is body strength, flexibility and durability that is obtained by weight training. The other is the health and viability of the heart, lungs and circulatory system that is built from aerobic training. There is minimal crossover effect between the two types of training. That is, if you lift weights you get some minimal positive effect on your cardiovascular system. Likewise, cardio training produces some minimal benefits for strength and durability. Thus, some cardio training is needed to build a fit body over 50.

10. **How much training do I have to do to get "fit"?** Doing basic lifting and cardio will help you achieve a foundation level of fitness for daily life. You don't have to become a powerlifter or a marathon runner to get huge benefits from being fit. In short, a little work done consistently over time will yield big benefits for your day to day life, and the overall quality of your life as you age into your 60's, 70's and beyond.   Having a foundation of fitness will significantly reduce your risk of contracting degenerative health conditions and debilitating chronic illness.

11. **Are there any supplements that will help make more rapid progress?** There is no substitute for regular training and good nutrition. People over 50 who try to find a short cut to success through using "supplements" are always disappointed in the results they get. They are also horrified at the price they must pay with unwanted side effects. Avoid performance enhancing drugs like the plague. They deliver little and extract a terrible price.

12. **How far can I go?** There is no way to tell in advance how far any individual can progress. There are some limits, but for the most part how far you progress is determined by your own dedication and hard work. Miraculous results are possible. They can be yours with work and perseverance.

Month

1

Program

"People tend to over estimate how much they can accomplish in one day and under estimate how much they can accomplish in a month"

-Steve Covey

"If you live easy, life is *hard*. If you live hard, life is easy."

-Pavel

Month 1: The Journey Begins

Start with Your vision

As you start getting back in shape, it is important to develop a vison of the person you want to become. What will you look like? How will it feel? What will be better than it is now?

Your vision motivates you to work hard and not backslide. It also gives you a way to chart your progress toward what you are trying to achieve.

Your vision is important because it motivates you for the training and nutrition actions you will be taking.

People who begin working out without a clear idea of what they want to accomplish will find that they have a lot of difficulty doing much of anything. Vague objectives such as "I only want to get toned", or "I want to lose a few pounds" lead nowhere as well.

An unclear vision leads to "drifting" or "being in the grey". There is no compelling reason to do something or not do something. Life just "happens".

Training without a clear vision is like getting in your car and starting to drive without any idea where you intend to go. If you said, "I'm going to Boston", you would select a route to that city and follow the path that takes you there. If you have no clear direction in mind, any direction is as good as any other.

Bottom line for you: develop a vision of what you want to accomplish with as much specificity as possible. Think about it every day. In aviation terminology, this will help keep you "on course, on glidepath".

Where are you starting?

Most people who begin this program will be in a de-conditioned state. It will have been at least a few years since they did regular physical exercise.

Don't be discouraged if you are in really poor condition.

Fitness is one of those rare areas in life where if you do the work, you are virtually guaranteed to be rewarded.

Some readers will have been doing some training but are not where they want to be.

Three things you should know:

- This course is the starting point for building up to levels of strength and health you may not be able to imagine right now. Everyone has to start at the foundation level.
- Where you start out in your fitness training has little impact on what you ultimately accomplish. Often those who are the least fit at the beginning are the ones who become the superstars.
- The most important element in success (as you will be reminded throughout this course) is *persistence!* Work hard, eat right, and keep your head on straight. You will be rewarded.

Already working out?

A few of you will already be doing some type of workout. If that is the case, good for you.

You may not be doing a comprehensive (weights and aerobics) program. Usually people do one or the other.

If you are already doing some weight training, do the exercises in this program, but can add some additional sets and reps if you are able to handle the workload. You also do the aerobic portion of the program.

Take the long view

Congratulations! It took guts to decide to get back into good condition.

You will have a far greater chance for success if you acknowledge that it will take time for you to reach the ideal vision you have set for yourself. You will see some nice results quickly, but real success comes in the long term.

Starting something new is easy. Staying with it until you succeed is hard. Anyone who tells you that you can go from de-conditioned to being in great shape in a few weeks is either a fool, a liar or both.

But, you will start feeling a bit better right away. Your body will be feasting on positive work and lots more oxygen than you are used to. You will start seeing and feeling results quickly.

The program in this book is designed to give you three months of solid training. You will make progress month after month. Once you have mastered the program in this book, I have multiple options for you to keep improving.

There are some ideas that will really help you sustain your commitment to building a fit and heathy body. I call these your "ecosystem of success".

Your Ecosystem of Success

"As a species, we should never underestimate our low tolerance for discomfort..."
-Pema Chodron, *The Places that Scare You*

That short quote sums up a lot of the reasons people quit fitness programs or any other activity that is difficult or unfamiliar.

If you want to dramatically enhance your chances for success, there are four areas that you should cultivate as your personal ecosystem of success.

- Understand the frustrations and discomfort you will confront
- Commit to your vision of what you want to achieve
- Surround yourself with positive energy and like-minded people
- Embrace a life of discovery

Understanding frustration and discomfort

"As a species, we should never underestimate our low tolerance for discomfort...."
-Pema Chodron *The Places that Scare You*

When things are predictable, there is no reason to fear them or feel uncomfortable. The person knows how events will unfold. They may still be 50 pounds overweight, but at least they "know" what it will feel like to follow their regular patterns. They won't have to confront the scary feelings that come up when they might have to deal with cutting out a meal!

When you take on a new set of activities, it is normal to feel such emotions as frustration, fear, pain, feeling unsafe, not knowing "the rules" that govern a new group, confusion, and so forth.

The reasons people quit fitness programs is usually that training takes them out of their "familiar zone". That is the pattern of life that they know well. They may not like parts of the pattern, but at least things are completely predictable in the familiar zone.

The eminent psychologist Kevin Hogan summarized the issue by noting that any time you start something new, you will encounter many frustrations and failures. One key to being successful is to understand that when you "feel" like you are failing, remind yourself that it is a "feeling" in your mind, _not reality_. Persist regardless of how you "feel".

When you feel frustrated or believe you are not making progress fast enough, don't take council of your fears or listen to excuses. Stick with the program and you will make progress toward your goal.

Quitting means success will never come.

Expect that a certain amount of frustration and discomfort will be part of achieving _anything_ that is worthwhile.

Commit to your vision

At age 50+ getting back in top physical condition may be the most important thing you do. Every day should re-commit to the vision you have of your future self.

Remember the quote by Steve Covey at the beginning of this section about how people over estimate what they can do in a day and under estimate what they can do in a month.

Getting fit does not happen in a simple linear manner. Your body will go through almost imperceptible changes each day, some of which you can see, and others less obvious.

It can be a big help if you keep a daily journal to track your progress. You can begin with a "selfie" and some measurements of your waist, chest, thigh, and arms. Also, record your body weight.

Think of becoming strong and fit as an _investment_ in yourself. When you do it, you get the dividends and benefits every day 24/7/365.

Having a strong vision of what you intend to accomplish will help sustain you when things get difficult. Keeping to a training program will get difficult at some point.

Surround yourself with positive energy and positive people

When you are trying to do something difficult, it is essential that you are supported by positive energy and positive associates around you.

You need to avoid or banish negative people from your life as much as possible.

Every person gives off either positive or negative energy (depending on the situation) and you need to be in a supportive and energizing environment. When training gets tough, it really helps when someone encourages you.

On the other hand, if you are trying to do something new and different (and difficult) there may be people around who will assure you that what you want to do is impossible. There always seems to be some "wise old owl" who has "seen everything" and "you will probably get injured or crippled from working out".

Banish this person from your life.

Others negativity comes from the fact that *they could not do* what you are attempting feel that your success would highlight their failure.

In direct contrast are those people who radiate positive energy and will do everything they can to encourage you. These are the people you need around you

Embrace a life of discovery

For some people, life has become nothing but a struggle from one unpleasant thing to another. There is nothing new or exciting.

 On the other hand, you are embarking on an *adventure* where you experience the joy of discovering how strong and fit you can become.

Your training sessions are where you rediscover your physicality, where you learn to do moves that you would have thought impossible before you started, and where you derive satisfaction from being able to do difficult things.

Training will be where you rediscover that "discipline is freedom". This is what every musician, artist, athlete, and successful person has practiced achieving what they desire.

You are embarking on a personal voyage of discovery.

Why People Quit Fitness Programs and Why You Wont

That short quote sums up most of the reasons people quit fitness programs, or any other activity that is difficult or unfamiliar.

How many people quit fitness programs? As noted earlier, in January each year millions of people head for fitness gyms armed with their new year's resolution to get in shape and probably lose weight. Of the new members who sign up *90% have quit within a month!!*

The reasons people quit fitness programs is usually that training takes them out of their "familiar zone". That is the pattern of life that they know well. They may not like parts of the pattern, but at least things are completely predictable in the familiar zone.

When things are predictable, there is no reason to fear them or feel uncomfortable. The person knows how events will unfold. They may still be 50 pounds overweight, but at least they "know" what it will feel like to follow their regular patterns. They won't have to confront the scary feelings that come up when they might have to deal with cutting out a meal!

When you take on a new set of activities, it is normal to feel such emotions as frustration, fear, pain, feeling unsafe, not knowing "the rules" that govern a new group, confusion, and so forth.

I won't lie to you and say that you won't confront some or all of these issues. Your eventual success will depend on how you manage your feelings around them.

If you stick with your training, over time all of the activities that were scary at first will become part of your "familiar zone". The gym will become part of "your turf".

But, achieving success will require that you overcome any (and all) of the fears and frustrations that come with starting something new and unfamiliar.

The eminent psychologist Kevin Hogan summarized the issue by noting that any time you start something new, you will encounter many frustrations and failures. The key to being successful will be to understand that when you fail or become frustrated, you persist regardless of how you "feel".

One of my own examples comes from 30+ years of riding horses. More than once I was deposited on the ground when the horse decided I was no longer needed on his back. At that point, you must "get back on the horse" or you will never become a competent rider.

When you feel frustrated or believe you are not making progress fast enough, don't take council of your fears or listen to excuses. Stick with the program and you will make progress toward your goal.

Quitting means success will never come.

I won't lie to you and tell you that physical training is *easy*. Anyone who does that is either stupid or a liar (or both). Getting physically fit is straightforward, but it is not easy.

Fitness is one of the areas of life where what you accomplish is almost directly related to how much effort and energy you put in.

You are already self-motivated and disciplined or you would never have bought this book. You just need to be aware that in the coming weeks and months your body and feelings will probably "fight back" against your determination to get fit.

Sticking with training despite all the difficulty will give you a deep feeling of satisfaction. You were one of the small number of people who had the guts, discipline, and determination to drive through difficulties and achieve your goal.

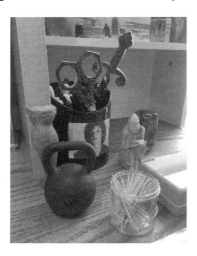

Month 1 Exercise Program

Weight training and Cardio training: Both are essential

Having radiant good health and fitness over age 50 requires all around conditioning. Being only strong or having superior endurance alone won't give you the health and longevity benefits you want.

I recognize that different people will prefer one type of training over another. There will be plenty of "gym rats" who can't wait to go lift iron. These people may not be nearly as enthusiastic about aerobic conditioning.

On the other hand, there will be the runners who can't wait to hit the trail. They may find lifting to be a chore.

Since I have done a lot of running and weight lifting, I can assure you that it is critical to do both if you want to get the body and health you want.

You need to do each of the routines 3 times a week with a day of rest between them. Any 3 days are fine.

You can do both types of training on the same day. I would recommend always doing the weight training first.

If some of the training is too hard for you at first, do what you can and continue to add more things as you get in better condition. Focus on improvement over time. Where you start is not as important as being persistent and consistent.

Weight training: Month 1

Getting back in condition to lift weights

We start by working to build your strength, mobility, and endurance.

Weight training will establish basic weight lifting movement patterns, developing a full range of motion, toughening up your muscles and connective tissues, and remind your body of all the fun you have when you lift weights.

All the weight exercises are multi-purpose. They focus not only on strength, but also on balance, coordination and full range of mobility.

Getting back full muscular coordination patterns means doing exercises that are compound movements. That means that many muscle groups must work together to do the exercise. In short, the exercises will emphasize *recruitment and coordination* rather than isolation.

The importance of using free weights.

A key emphasis in this course is developing athleticism as well as strength and overall fitness. Because of this I strongly suggest doing only a few carefully selected machine-based exercises.

A well-conditioned body has muscles that work together in a coordinated manner. Free weights require that your whole body works together to do a lift. *If you use weight machines, you get near zero benefit for coordination, athleticism, or stability.* The machine does all that work for you, and thus robs you of much of the benefit you could get from exercising.

In the words of a friend of mine who is a Russian Master of Sport, "machines will suck the athleticism right out of you".

With very few exceptions, I include mainly exercises *done with free weights while standing on your feet!*

There are exceptions to this...the bench press lat pull down, and incline press being most notable. However, my 60+ years of training have convinced me that with few exceptions, weight machines don't give you much help in your quest to get in excellent condition.

Mental Focus and Improving Performance

These days I see people "training" in gyms while they watch television, listen to music in their headsets, or have an intense "relationship" with their cell phone.

I observe that these same people rarely improve much beyond the first few months of training. Many of them have astonishingly poor lifting technique. They "flop and thrash" through different exercises and probably wonder why they don't get better.

Being distracted by either technology or conversation means their mind is "somewhere else" during the training session. IMHO this means that whatever training they are doing is largely wasted. When you are not concentrating completely on what you are doing, little progress is possible.

If you are going to succeed at reconditioning your body, it is essential that you devote all your attention and focus to what you are doing. That means ditch the "entertainment" and most of the socializing during workouts. You should concentrate on the movements you are doing.

In weight training this means you should be focusing on doing every repetition correctly. This means you should be "feeling" what it is like to do a perfect rep. You should also be fully aware of what your body is doing during an exercise. That way you will build strength, coordination, and athleticism.

When you are doing aerobic training, you should be "feeling" your body in coordinated motion. You should never "tune out". You should be aware of your breathing and cadence. You should be conscious of how each part of your body feels as you speed up or slow down. In short, toss the ear buds and music player and concentrate on what is happening with YOU.

Your focus and concentration will play a bigger and bigger role in making progress the longer you train. Developing powerful focus takes practice. It is a great idea to start doing this right from the first day you start training.

Weight training exercises: Month 1

Schedule

Month 1 weight training in will be done as follows:

- Train 3 days a week with at least one day in between
- Take 60-90 seconds between sets of an exercise
- Recover fully between exercises

Week 1-2:

- Do **2 sets of 6 repetitions**.
- Increase the weight by 5 pounds when the second set is easy to do
- Recover fully between sets and between exercises

Week 3-4:

- Do **2 sets of 8 repetitions**
- Increase the weight by 5 pounds when the second set is easy to do
- Take no more than 2 minutes between sets or between exercises

Month 1

Exercises

1. Standing dumbbell press (2 sets x 6-8 reps)
2. One arm rowing (2 x 6-8)
3. Kettlebell/dumbbell swing (2 x 6-8)
4. Bench press (2 x 6-8)
5. Dumbbell curl (2 x 6-8)
6. Unweighted squat (2 x 6-8)
7. Suitcase deadlift (2 x 6-8)
8. Plank (15-60 seconds)

Terminology

Whole Body Lift – These are lifts that literally involve every muscle in the body. These are always compound movements that involve moving a heavy weight.

Getting maximum performance doing a whole-body lift requires focus on activating all muscle groups that need to be involved. When the lift has been mastered, activation of all the various muscle groups should be second nature.

Whole body lifts used in this course include the following:
- Squat
- Bench Press
- Deadift
- Overhead presses
- Kettlebell swings
- Front squats
- Power Cleans

Recruiting muscles – To develop maximum power, it is essential to activate every muscle in your body during a lift. This is particularly true for whole body lifts but applies to other lifts as well.

Recruiting requires that every muscle be tensed during performance of a lift. For example, when doing a squat, it is necessary to ensure that every muscle group in the body is tense before beginning the descent. If any muscle group is relaxed, it is like having a leak in a hydraulic system. All the pressure in the system moves toward leak and the system collapses toward the leak.

This is the exact opposite of the idea of *isolation* which is a bodybuilding practice where the lifter attempts to focus all the work done in an exercise on one muscle group. Isolation undercuts any chance a lifter might have to build serious strength. It can also create a dangerous situation where a lifter can lose control of a heavy weight.

---

1. Standing dumbbell press

The standing press is one of the greatest exercises ever devised. It can not only be a good test of strength, but it requires mobilization of many sets of muscles to do the movement. It is what is known as a *whole-body exercise.*

You can do this with either dumbbells or kettlebells. The training effect is basically the same.

Begin by standing upright with your feet slightly wider than shoulder width. Bring the weights to your shoulders to the starting press position.

At this point *tighten your entire body.* Tighten your legs, lock your knees, dig your toes into the floor, pinch your glutes together, tighten your abs, and your neck. Then *squeeze the dumbbell (or kettlebell) handle hard!*

Every muscle in your body should be tight. There should *never* be any muscles that are relaxed. You are now locked tight ready to do an overhead press.

Take a deep breath and hold it.

Drive the weight in your right hand upward so that it is next to your head. When it is above your head, push slightly back so that when your arm is fully extended, the weight is directly over your head.

When the weight in your right hand is over head at arm's length, release your breath and lower the weight under control to the starting point.

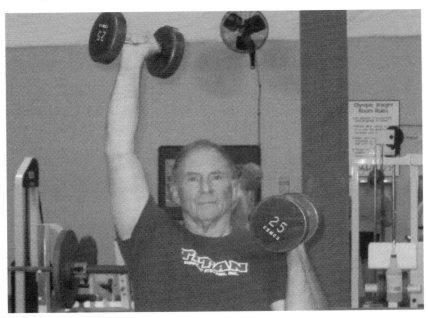

Standing dumbbell press – Alternating hands

Now, repeat the lift with your left hand. When this is done, do the next rep with the right hand.

You should do 6 (or 8) repetitions *with each hand.*

The overhead press will condition not only your shoulders, triceps, and upper back, but your abdominals, and all the other stabilizer muscles in your body.

You will also be building the skill of *recruiting* muscles to do heavy lifting. This will be a critical athletic skill in building strength. **Two sets of 6-8 repetitions.**

2. One arm rowing

The next exercise is the one arm rowing motion. This primarily conditions the latissimus (back)

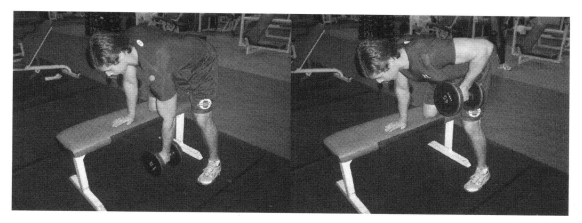

One arm rowing: starting position and top position

Begin by putting your left knee on a bench or chair. Then put your left hand down on the bench. Hold the weight in your right hand at arm's length.

Your back should be flat, your abs tight (not sucked in) and your head should be slightly up.

Tighten your body as much as you can, take a deep breath and hold it, then bring the weight up to your waist. Pause, then slowly lower it to the starting position while gradually releasing your breath.

After you have done 6-8 repetitions move the weight to your left hand and, do the rowing exercise with the right knee and hand on the bench.

When you have done 6-8 reps with both your left and right hands, you have done one set.

An alternate way to do this is to brace yourself by putting your left hand on your left knee (and the reverse). The main idea is to brace yourself on the opposite side from where you are pulling the weight and keep tight.

You will do **2 sets of 6-8 repetitions** with each arm.

3. Kettlebell/dumbbell swing

The Russian or Hard Style swing is the foundation for the spectacular conditioning routines that are done with kettlebells. In my opinion, this exercise should be part of every workout program you do as long as you train.

With that subdued introduction, let me show you the kettlebell swing that will be part of your reconditioning program.

You begin by doing the two-hand version of the swing. In the third month you will begin using the one hand version. Both are great conditioning movements.

Begin standing erect with your feet a slightly wider than shoulder width. The weight will be on the floor in front of you.

With your back flat, bend your knees and go down to grasp the kettlebell handle with both hands. Take a deep breath, tense your abs and swing the kettlebell back between your legs as if you were hiking a football.

Keep your back flat and head up as you swing the weight back between your legs.

When the weight is as far back as it will go, drive your hips forward explosively and straighten your knees. Keep your arms against your body as the weight is driven upward. Keep the back flat.

Your arms should do nothing to move the weight upward. All the force comes from your hip drive, your glutes, and tight abs. As you near the point where your arms are parallel to the floor, you should lean back slightly and exhale quickly. Your glutes and abdominal muscles should be fully flexed at the top of the swing.

When the weight has reached a point where your arms are parallel to the ground (or slightly above), it should "float" for a split second before gravity kicks in and it starts back down.

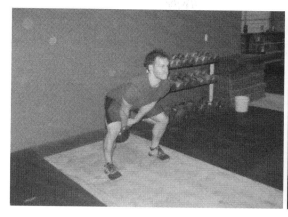 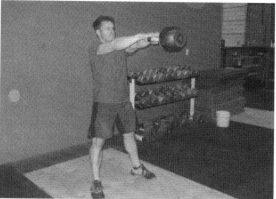

Weight behind in "hike" position   Top of the swing

You should quickly inhale (and hold it) just as the weight begins to descend. You allow the weight to swing back between your legs, and then explosively reverse the thrust. Your drive out of the bottom will be done holding your breath with fully tensed abs.

You should feel the main exertion of the swing in the glutes, hamstrings and abs. If you feel a lot in your lower back, you are probably bending over too far and need to position your shoulders back so that they are over your knees when you start the swing.

In this first month you will be mastering the technique of the swing. You will be doing **2 sets of 6-8 reps.**

4. Bench Press

Perhaps the most popular gym lift in the present time, bench pressing is deceptively difficult to do well. We will focus on correct body mechanics for a good bench, and work on reconditioning shoulders for heavy lifting.

As some of you have trained previously, it is highly probable that you did the bench press. Unless you trained with competitive power lifters, there is a 98% chance that your bench press technique was deficient in some way.

Poor technique means that you probably did the lift in a way that will prevent you from coming anywhere near to your full potential. Your long-term objective is to get as strong and fit as possible. Thus, excellent lifting technique is mandatory.

The first rule of bench pressing is that this is a *whole-body lift.* You are going to learn how to mobilize every muscle in your body to get a good bench press.

You begin by getting your whole body tight. Successful bench pressing involves *recruiting* every muscle you can. Just the opposite of isolation.

You should begin by getting into proper position on the bench.

As you can see in the pictures below, the feet are placed so that the heels are well behind the knees. This will enhance tightness in the back. Your butt is on the bench, and there is a tight arch in your lower back.

Your shoulders are firmly in contact with the bench. Your shoulders should be pushed down toward the toes.

The grip spacing will vary by individual, but the most common one is wider than shoulder width.

When you are set up on the bench, you should squeeze the bar with your hands, and try to bend the bar as you hold it. This will activate muscles throughout your body.

Lift the bar off the rack, and it should be in a position right over your face.

Take a deep breath and hold it.

Slowly lower the bar to the top of your stomach, or the bottom of your rib cage, (not the middle of your chest).

As you lower the bar, bring your elbows in toward your sides. This will activate your back muscles for the push out of the bottom.

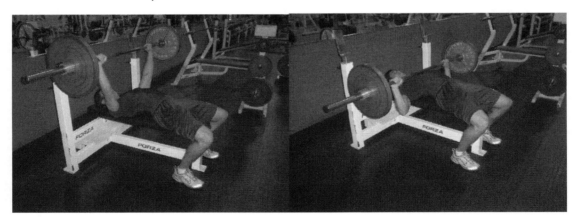

Starting Position   Bar on Chest ready to press

When the bar touches your chest at the point described above, pause briefly, and drive the bar back to the starting position.

When the bar is about ¾ of the way back to the starting position, you can release your breath.

Take in another deep breath and hold it before you lower the bar again.

You should do **2 sets of 6-8 reps**.

Keep the weights light, you will find that your strength will build rapidly if you do not exert more than 80% effort on any one rep.

5. Dumbbell biceps curl

The biceps curl is one of the most popular exercises in all of weightlifting. The reason is that it produces great looking arms. As such it is one of the "t-shirt" exercises.

In addition to building a great "look", the curl builds strength in your biceps, forearms, hands and shoulders.

There are many variations of the curl, and the dumbbell version is a great one to use at the start of your re-conditioning training.

Take a dumbbell in each hand with your arms straight down at your sides. Your palms should be facing out at the start of the movement.

Bring the dumbbell in your right hand up to your right shoulder by bringing your forearm up. Your elbow can be braced against your side, or slightly ahead of your body and palm facing upward as you curl the bell to your shoulder.

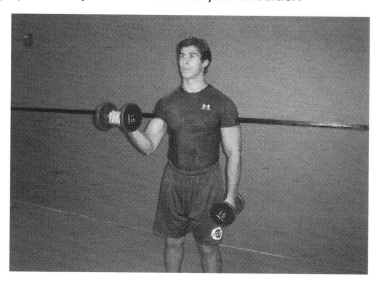

Alternate dumbbell curl

In this exercise you will do one rep with the right hand and then one rep with the left. Do that until you have done 6-8 reps with each hand.

It is important that you begin with a weight that is light enough so that you can do the exercise *entirely* with your biceps. You should not use any other body motion to move the weight.

It is also important that you begin each repetition with your arm *straight*. If the arm is bent you do not use the full range of motion for building the muscle.

Do **2 sets of 6-8 reps.**

6. Unweighted squats

Most people who have been out of training for an extended period find that their leg power has diminished significantly. This takes two forms: 1) peak power has diminished; and 2) many muscles are strong only in very limited range of motion.

It is to be expected that peak power will diminish. However, in my experience, the most common problem for reconditioning is that support muscles needed to do *deep squats* have deteriorated to an even greater degree than other muscles.

This is particularly true of the muscles on the inside of the thigh, the hip flexors and those in the lower back. All these muscles to be reconditioned or you risk getting injured.

For this reason, I begin reconditioning with unweighted squats where the intent is to build up the full range of squat motion and begin to bring unused muscles back up to the level where it is possible to train with intensity again.

Our objective is to get your leg muscles back into shape to do regular squats.

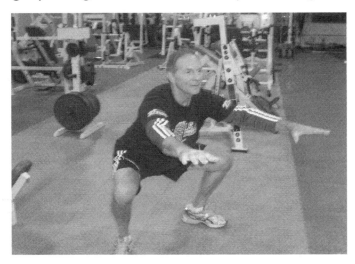

Unweighted Squat

The unweighted squat begins standing fully erect, feet should be roughly 3 inches wider than your shoulders (15 cm) on each side, and hands either out in front, or at your sides.

Take a deep breath and hold it. Descend by sitting back as if you were going to be seated in a chair. Keep your chest up throughout the squat. Your weight will be on your heels, but your toes should dig into the floor for stability and activating all your leg muscles.

You should try to keep your shins as vertical as possible. In any event, never allow your knees to get out ahead of a line coming straight up from your toes.

In your first training sessions concentrate on going as deep as you can without pain. If you experience pain, go easy and see what you can do comfortably.

You should do squats **2 sets of 6-8 repetitions**

Initially you may find that you are stiff and cannot do a full squat. Over a period of days or weeks you may be able to become more flexible and eventually get so that you can do a deep squat.

Many over age 50 bodies have accumulated physical "damage" from life. Much of it can be reversed or managed. Some you can do yourself, others may require help from a sports medicine professional.

If you find that you cannot progress beyond a certain point without pain, you should consult a physical therapist to see what can be done to restore your flexibility.

In no event should you force yourself to do squat movements when pain either persists or gets worse.

7. Dumbbell or Kettlebell "Suitcase" Deadlift

Deadlifting is one of the best "whole body" exercises ever devised. You will be doing barbell deadlifts in the coming months.

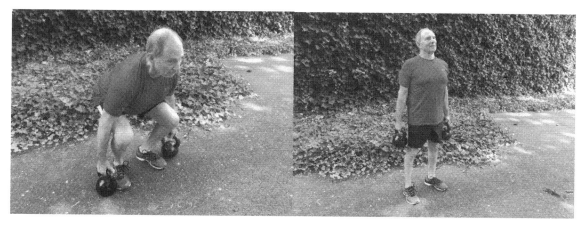

Dumbbell Deadlift – Start   Dumbbell Deadlift - Finish

In the first month deadlifting will be done with light weights held to the side of your body. The emphasis will be on reestablishing your flexibility and range of motion.

The proper starting and finishing positions for the suitcase deadlift are shown in the pictures above.

It is critical to do the deadlift with proper technique. Your back must be flat and hips low throughout this exercise. You will be pulling and lowering the weights by bending your legs and tensing your abdominal muscles. Keep your hips down and lift by "pushing" with the legs. You should *never* raise and lower the weights by simply bending over at the waist.

Good technique is not simply for aesthetics or "style points". Good technique is necessary to generate full pulling power, get the most benefit from the movement, and drastically limit the likelihood of injury.

Ideally you should be able to grasp two dumbbells or kettlebells that are sitting on the floor (or ground) a few inches from each foot. If you have been out of training for a while, you may not have the flexibility to get into the starting position easily.

If you can't get down to grasp the weights, you can begin holding the weights while standing erect. Then lower yourself down until the weights touch the floor. Use weights that are relatively light for you until you are comfortably able to begin with the weights on the floor. Then you can be more ambitious with the weight you use.

Your heels should be 12-18 inches apart. (30-45 cm). It is best if you wear shoes without a raised heel as this tends to push you forward more than is optimal.

The technique shown here will allow you to re-develop your pulling power and get your body accustomed to the full range of the deadlift movement without using much weight.

If you have not lifted for many months (or years), you should begin with very light weights. Don't increase the weights until you find a weight that is easy for the first four reps and only mildly difficult for the last two.

Eventually you will most likely be able to pull huge weights in the deadlift. In this phase of reconditioning focus on getting into the start position, rebuilding your posterior power train, correcting specific weaknesses or muscle imbalances.

Do **2 sets of 6-8 reps.**

8. Abdominal Plank

Building your core strength is one of the most important things you can do for having good health and quality of life. Core strength is critical for preventing chronic conditions such as back pain, leg pain and knee pain from emerging as you age.

You will need a timer for this exercise as you will be doing it for a specific number of seconds. An inexpensive stop watch will work well, or the sweep second hand on any available clock. There are many options.

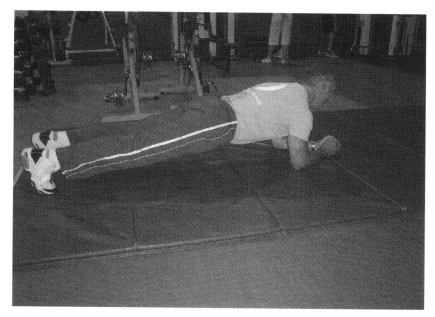

Begin by getting on the floor as if you were going to do pushups. Rest your weight on your forearms and your toes. Raise your hips up until all your weight is resting on your forearms and toes. Keep your back straight and don't allow your rear end to go up in the air.

You hold the position shown in the photo for 10-30 seconds. Work up to the point where you can hold the plank position 2 times for at least 30 seconds.

That concludes the resistance training part of the workout. Now for the aerobics.

Month 1 Aerobic training

Aerobic Training: Month 1

For people over age 50 it is difficult to know their level of aerobic fitness if they have not worked out for a long time. If someone is overweight it is particularly risky to begin a program without first getting a doctor's clearance to train.

Aerobic fitness is critical to reduce the risk of heart attack or stroke. Aerobic training has also been linked to a significant reduction in the chances for developing dementia. In combination with weight training, aerobics can help anyone over age 50 build a healthy, resilient, and powerful body.

In this program, I'm going to present some options that the reader can use depending on their current level of aerobic fitness.

It is important to understand that in all physical training, it is impossible to predict how fit you can become based on your starting condition. People can be severely out of shape and build up phenomenal levels of fitness if they do the work and persevere.

If someone is out of shape, even former athletes, it may take months to get back to a foundation level of fitness. It is critical not to be impatient. Start with the basics and work up.

You should clearly understand that the primary purpose of aerobic training is to revitalize your cardiovascular system, NOT LOSE FAT.

Cardio training for fat loss is minimally effective because: 1) you must be in good condition to do enough training to burn much fat; and 2) as you get in better shape, you use fewer and fewer calories to do the same amount of cardio work. But, more on this in later sections.

There are some HUGE benefits that come from even modest amounts of aerobic training that are not widely discussed. One of the most important ones is that *aerobic training improves brain function and helps reduce the chances of dementia.*

Options for aerobic training

There are multiple options for doing aerobics training. These include jogging, walking, cycling, rowing, swimming, stair climbing, etc.

You select one you like, or dislike the least, and do 5-10 minutes of movement at a slow steady pace. This is the "minimum dose" that will get you back on the road to being in good condition.

Gradually increase the time you do aerobics as you feel stronger. In the first month, don't exceed 15 minutes if you are just getting back in condition.

In the coming months aerobic training will become more demanding. If you are starting in a deconditioned state, you should focus on getting regular movement, and beginning the process of reconditioning your heart, lungs, and circulatory system.

You should do aerobic training 3 times a week.

Remember, the goal is to enhance your stamina, and build up your heart, lungs, and circulatory system. It is NOT to prepare you to run a marathon (or even a 5K).

Running may not be a good idea if you weigh over 200 lbs. (90 Kilos). Your knees, hips, feet, etc. may not benefit from the pounding.

LOW impact will protect the joints, muscles, and connective tissues.

This program should be done at an easy pace that gets your heart working at a slightly elevated but steady level. The benefit comes from circulating a lot of oxygen rich blood to all your muscles and internal organs.

Why do I suggest a 10-minute maximum for this program in the first month? I want to minimize the reasons for you to avoid aerobics training and minimize the chance for injury.

Remember, about 90% of the people who start a new fitness program will quit within 30 days. One reason for quitting is that the program is too difficult, or it takes "too much time".

Whichever form of aerobics training you choose, _the most important thing is to select something you will actually do on a consistent basis._

You get no benefit from a great program that you don't do.

Starting slow

Some of you who are reading this book will already be doing some aerobic training. A few of you may already be doing demanding aerobic training. If this is the case, continue doing what you are already doing, but add the weight training workouts to your program.

For people who are not doing aerobics training, your reconditioning program will begin at a very low intensity.

There are multiple reasons for this. Many people over age 50 can have a substantially diminished cardiovascular capacity. Even though it can be rebuilt, it is imperative that it be done gradually.

Another reason to begin gradually is that it will take a while for your body's muscles, joints, and connective tissues to adapt to aerobic training.

In short, start with low intensity and short duration. Gradually build up as your cardiovascular system and your body get in better condition.

Aerobic Level 1

The most important thing to do in aerobics reconditioning is to get the heart rate up from resting pulse rate and keep it there for 10-15 minutes.

There are multiple options for aerobic training. These are walking, running, cycling, swimming, treadmill or stair climber, stationary bicycle, rowing machine, etc.

The choice is up to you.

It is necessary to do aerobic training at least three times a week every week during the first month.

It is also important that if you are beginning in a completely deconditioned state that you select a training option that is *low impact*. The best way to avoid injuries that come when starting back is to work back into training gradually and minimize the shock to your system.

If you are overweight it is particularly important not to begin with running or jogging until you have done a few weeks of walking. Your body will not be used to the shocks and jarring of running and you don't want injuries to slow your progress.

Aerobic Level 2

If you have already been doing some aerobic training, you will not need to start from scratch. You should begin training using your present program.

This applies whether you are running, cycling, rowing, swimming, etc.

Over the coming weeks you will gradually increase the volume and intensity of the aerobic training you do.

Always remember that "train, don't strain" is the best guidance for how much you should do. The purpose of this program is to build up steadily and gradually.

Being wise about how much training you do is part of the using your mind to build your body.

Being Present and Improving Performance

Earlier I talked about being present and aware to help reconnect you with the physical world. Being present is also essential if you want to improve your performance in lifting or aerobics.

You have no doubt seen people in a gym, or on a home treadmill, watching television or listening to music while they do their work out. They are "living in their heads" not in their bodies when they do this.

If you are going to rebuild your body, *it is essential that you be <u>fully aware</u> of what you are doing all the time while you are training.* You want to use training time to do the work and *teach your body how to do the training correctly.*

Most people lifting weights in a gym have poor (or atrocious) form. Realizing your full potential requires excellent form. Eliminate distractions and focus on doing each rep correctly and learning exactly what it feels like to do the movement correctly. Let other people "flop and thrash" their way through a workout.

I'm going to strongly suggest that you *never* have any distraction while you work out. Forget the headset and iPhone. You should concentrate fully on how you feel, on your breathing, on the sensation in your arms and legs, etc.

There is nothing you could be doing for the 10-15 minutes of aerobics that is nearly as important as being aware of your body and getting the "feel" of moving. You are learning how to control your movements in ways you may never have thought about before.

Month 1: Nutrition

Basic Approach to Nutrition

I operate on the theory that it is much easier to focus on a few key things and get them right, rather than trying to do a dozen different things. For that reason, each month I'll introduce a few key ideas that you can work on.

In my view, focusing on a certain "diet" is a mistake because that while it may lead to some fat loss, the real issue for many people is that they have some *habits* (habitual patterns of doing things) that need to be changed. Once the habits have been changed, much of the extra fat drops away.

Why no "diet"?

Most people who want to "get back into shape" need to lose *some* body fat.   Based on my casual (unscientific) survey of seeing people in stores, offices, airports, etc. my guess is that most folks have a little extra "table muscle". Some have a *lot* extra, but I'll get to them later.

Most fat loss diets appear to begin with the idea that you are an idiot that needs hundreds of rules on what to eat and not eat, or you will "hog out" every time you pass a mini-mart.

While this may be true for some people, most people will get a huge benefit from simply changing a *few habits*. Once this is done, they will tend to eat in a way that is right for them.

There are literally hundreds of "diets" out there. Some of them work OK and others work for about a week.

Starting a diet is easy. Most people can stay on one for a few days or weeks. Then things get difficult. A lot of unplanned temptations keep popping up. The stress of constantly denying things the dieter may really "want" can become overwhelming.

Strict diets do appear to help people get rid of excess fat, even a lot of it. *What they fail to do is help the person keep the weight off* for more than a week or two.

There are many stories about people who have dropped 100 pounds and then within a year gained all of it back plus another 10-20 pounds.

In a recent study of contestants of the popular television show *The Biggest Looser*, researchers found that after six years the contestants had regained and average of 90% of the fat they lost.

In cases like this it is obvious that while staying on a diet can result in fat loss, the diet is not solving the real problem. Many people who become obese are often fighting mental and emotional issues that lead to compulsive eating.

Most (if not all) people will benefit from focusing their energy on developing healthy habits.

Exercise Alone won't lead to significant fat loss

If you are starting back on an exercise program, and you are carrying anywhere from 10-50 "extra" pounds (aka. "fat"), simply working out again is going to have minimal impact on your "table muscle".

Some people believe that since they are no longer sedentary, the fat will drop off because they are training again. Reality is that you will probably lose some fat, but that will happen in the early going when your body is getting used to the shock of you working out again.

Getting lean will require that you eat less. In some cases, a lot less. It all depends on how much you currently consume.

As you become aware of how much you are actually eating, you should be making some adjustments in your consumption right away. Cutting out a lot of unplanned eating may have a big impact or minimal impact. It depends on how much you were eating before starting on this program.

There are a variety of expensive tech gadgets available that imply that they can help you get fit. They count the steps you take or give an estimate of the calories you burn doing different activities, or something else that it is easy for a wearable tech gadget to measure.

IMHO these devices are pretty much useless. They will tend to give you a lot of data that is either unimportant or inaccurate. For example, counting steps during the day is of minimal value if you are doing even a modest amount of training. The number of calories burned by a given exercise will vary widely from one person to another.

Counting steps is trivial when compared to monitoring how much you eat each day.

An inexpensive digital monitor can't provide *truly important* measures of fitness such as improved coordination, improved muscle activation by the central nervous system, increased cardiovascular fitness, or changes in muscle density.

So, forget the gadgets or toss them in the trash.

Simple Decision Rules

If you need to drop a significant amount of fat (10-50 pounds or more), you will have to take serious action to reduce your food intake.

I would recommend that you begin by cutting your food intake 20-25% across the board. Some will argue that this is too drastic.

My response is *that if you want to cut from 225 lbs to 175 lbs. you are going to have to eat like a fit 175-pound person.* At that size you will normally eat a lot less than if you weighed 225. In short, if you want to be a 175-pound athlete, eat like one and that is what you will gradually become.

In my view, one of the biggest problem people have in *staying on* a diet program face is *having to make a lot of "decisions" about what to eat every day.* If you must "decide" what to eat every time you are confronted with a meal or snack opportunity, you will routinely find a reason to make a poor choice. Eventually, the diet goes out the window because it takes too much effort.

For this reason, I recommend that you begin your program by adopting a strategy that will help you lose fat and build muscle.

What this approach does is *eliminate the need to <u>make choices</u> every time a tempting situation comes up.* If someone offers you a chocolate chip cookie during your fasting period, the answer is a simple "no thanks".

One of the reasons that this approach works is that *it takes all the ambiguity* out of any situation where you are presented an opportunity to eat.

By eliminating the "decision" to eat or not, you minimize the amount of "discipline" that will be needed to manage your eating.

After a short period of adjustment, you will probably find that this approach is relatively easy to maintain indefinitely.

Basic Habits for Eating right

These changes can have a huge impact on your overall health and will help you build muscle and lose fat.

In the first month of this program you should focus on making five changes in your nutrition:

1. Eat fresh unprocessed food
2. Eliminate junk from your eating

3. Stop "mindless" eating
4. Cut out as much sugar as feasible
5. Drink plenty of water

Eat Fresh Food

Processed food is typically loaded with extra sugar, salt and fat to make it more palatable. For this reason, it will taste good, but will make you fat and unhealthy.

Begin your fitness transformation by avoiding processed food (anything in a bag or can). This includes all "chips", most "dips", processed meats (hot dogs, sausages, "lunch meat" etc.), canned fruit and vegetables (extra sugar), packaged desserts, processed cheese, crackers, cookies, sweet rolls, and so on.

Select your groceries from the fresh produce section, fresh meat and fish, fresh dairy products, and fresh frozen products.

Rather than give you a laundry list of products to avoid, you should begin focusing on general types of things that are good for you to eat.   This strategy will be of great value to you as you go forward in your reconditioning program.

Don't eat Crap

It can be said that for most crap food, you don't need to put it in your mouth, you can just apply it directly to your ass.

There is a lot of edible material for sale these days that humans can digest, but it is not good for someone who wants to be fit and healthy.   These "food like" items are offered for sale in places like coffee shops, mini-marts, gas stations, vending machines, big box stores and perhaps even in a few select funeral parlors.

Some of these items masquerade as "health food" by focusing on a minor ingredient whose positive effect is swamped by the ton of bad stuff. Among the chief offenders are things like "bran muffins", "breakfast sandwiches", "fat-free cookies", "energy drinks", "doughnuts" and countless others.

Some crap foods are made from "organic" sources. That does not make them any less crap.

Major ingredients in these diabolical preparations are white flour, fat, sugar, and salt. Added fat, salt and sugar are used in lavish amounts to make the food more appealing, and addicting.

Some of these preparations are marketed as "natural". Just remember some of the deadliest poisons are "natural" elements: arsenic, lead, cobalt, etc. Saying a food is "natural" is basically a pointless marketing slogan.

The types of crap that are most common are "chips", comfort foods such as desserts, snack foods, and candy.

Among the most sinister products that you should avoid like the plague are "energy drinks" and "sports drinks". Most are simply sugar and caffeine with little or no nutritional value.

Step one in the nutrition part of your reconditioning should be to educate yourself on the vast array of junk available for consumption. Once educated, you should systematically purge it from your regular eating.

Mindless eating

One habit that will really help you gain control of your health and fitness is the practice of being *conscious* of everything you eat.

Most people will say, "of course I'm aware of what I eat". But, think about this scenario.

You go to a meeting at work, and someone brings doughnuts. Without thinking, you take one along with most of your co-workers.

Here is another common occurrence. You are watching television and a bag of chips appears. You "graze" on these for a while during the show.

Yet another time when unplanned and unconscious eating occurs.

You stop for gas on a road trip and buy a few "snacks" at the mini-mart inside the gas station. The munching "helps pass the time" while you drive.

The common thread in all of these situations is that you would probably not have eaten any of these things (all of them junk) if you thought ahead. They simply appeared in your path and you took them because it was easy.

The cumulative effect of these easy eating opportunities may be residing around your waistline or on your butt. They may also have given you some unwanted medical conditions such as high blood pressure or a pre-diabetic condition.

The net effect of unconscious eating can be really damaging.

Your biggest defense against this is to *not have it in your house*.

Sugar: Your mortal enemy

Sugar is used as an additive in more foods than you can count. This is because it tastes good. A little sugar is good for you. A lot is really bad for you. Most people eat a lot more than they should.

In the first month of your reconditioning program, you need to be aggressive in finding all the overlooked or ignored sources of sugar in your daily diet and eliminate them.

You should make it a practice to read food labels on every can and package of stuff you put in your mouth during this first month. You will be stunned to find that sugar is mixed into many things you would never suspect.

Your body makes no distinction between the sugar hidden in food products from sugar consumed as sugar. It all goes into your system for processing. Extra sugar gets stored as fat.

When you root out the "stealth" sugar in your diet, you will find that you drop a few pounds without making any other changes.

Sugar is mildly addicting and is not always easy to quit. Be aware that your body may fight back when you try to reduce your sugar consumption.

By getting rid of unwanted sugar, you can eat sugar *when you make a choice to do so.*

Water is a magic liquid

Drinking 8-10 8-ounce glasses of water throughout the day will help your body in many ways. It will facilitate digestion of your food, enhance your metabolism, help burn fat, help prevent muscle cramps, and maintain your electrolyte balance for mental sharpness.

For helping maintain a fit body, there is no liquid you can drink that beats water.

Drinking water is one of those situations where some people appear believe that if a little is good, then an enormous amount must be great. I recall the story from about fifteen years ago about two runners in a big marathon race who actually killed themselves by drinking too much water (destroyed their electrolyte balance).

Water consumption is one of those areas where people can get stupid and guzzle gallons of water when modest amounts are good. Just make certain you drink what you need every day.

You are the boss (of what goes into your mouth)

You are "in charge" of your eating. That is the good news and the bad news.

In the first month you need *to become <u>fully aware</u> of what you are eating.*

When you *decide* to eat chips or a mocha latte' it is a *choice* you made, not simply something that you do on autopilot.

You will also be working on establishing a "new normal" for your eating.

If you have extra fat, the way you ate in the past is a big reason you are in your present condition.

For some people making changes in eating habits will be difficult. For others, not so much. The key to long term success is to eliminate bad habits and develop good ones.

Month 1: Motivation and Mindset

If getting in great shape was easy, everyone would have a perfect body. It is not easy, but it is one of those rare things that if you do the work, you can literally feel the payoff 24/7/365.

As you begin physical training again it is critical to understand that the powerful role your mindset plays in of whether you succeed or fail. You are attempting to make a big change in your life, and how you think about what you are attempting drives what you do.

I'll remind you over and over that 90% of the people who begin an exercise program will quit at some point in the first month. Much of the reason for this is what they are thinking.

One of my most important tasks in this first month is to help you understand how mindset can either be a big asset in your quest for fitness, or the thing that makes you part of the 90% who quit.

I don't think that most people begin a fitness program believing they are going to fail. But I do think that many begin believing many _reasons_ *why they are going to fail.*

On the other hand, there are people who mobilize the power of their mind to generate success in new and complex undertakings. This is where you want to be.

Let's look at how to use your mind to help you get the best results.

The "fixed" mindset

Why do people avoid doing something they know would be good for them?

One of the things that I believe stops many people in their tracks *is not believing they can do something.* Each of us have ideas in our mind that create our *personal reality.* These are things we *believe* but are not necessarily *true.* These ideas can cause us a lot of problems.

First are the expectations that people have when they begin a program. Many people will begin a fitness program *unconsciously expecting to fail!*

If you asked them, they would never say "I don't think I can do this", but in their mind many doubts abound. These will take the form of ideas such as: "I have never been a good athlete", "My body type will keep me from looking good", "I just want to get toned", or "People in great condition over 50 are just naturals".

These ideas, and variations on them, conspire to limit the chances of someone's success before they even start work.

This is called a *fixed* mindset. It means that people *believe* they can *determine in advance* how successful they will be at any endeavor.

Some common examples of a fixed mindset are: "I could never learn to dance, I'm too clumsy", "I'm no good at math", "I'm not very smart", "I'm not athletic at all", "I'm naturally fat", "I'm a looser", "this is way too hard for someone like me", and so on.

The common theme in all these *ideas* is that the person *thinks* they can tell in advance how successful they will be at something *before they try to do it!*

People with fixed mindsets accept huge limitations on their potential *before* they even try to do something.

The "Growth Mindset"

The good news is that researcher Dr. Carol Dweck has shown that in most things ***it is impossible to predict in advance how successful someone can be at a task, if they work at it.***

This is called the ***growth mindset.*** It means that one will only find out how successful they can be by working persistently at something.

People who have a growth mindset take on a new task believing "It will be difficult, but I can do this", "there will be times when I want to quit", "if I have a bad day, I'll do better next time", "all this work is worth it", "I'm improving every day", "I feel good about myself for doing this" and so forth.

When you have a growth mindset you approach the task knowing it may be difficult, but you are committed to giving it your best shot.

In the coming months I'll emphasize the liberating power of the growth mindset and how it can bring great things to your life in fitness and in almost any area you choose.

For now, in terms of *your* physical fitness, realize that there is *no way to tell in advance* how strong, agile, resilient, and capable you can become. That is to be determined by your hard work and persistence.

How far you can go can *only to be discovered through persistent work.*

The power of "a plan"

As the legendary powerlifter Bull Stewart said often, *"if you have no plan, your plan is to fail!"*

When people have no plan, they will simply be *drifting.* Daily circumstances will push them one way one day and another direction the next. Life just "happens" to them.

But…YOU have a plan. Your exercise and nutrition plan is the one in this book.

Every month you will be using this plan to master more skills of being fit.

How you go about *doing* those things is determined by your mindset and motivation.

It is easy to make plans, and then ignore them. That is what a lot of people do.

You must assert that *you are in control* of what goes on in your life. To get back in shape you must *assert control over your exercise and nutrition.*

You must *recommit every day* that you will follow the exercise and nutrition program in this book.

The Power of Persistence

One of my favorite quotes of all time sums up the overwhelming power of being persistent.

> "Nothing in the world can take the place of Persistence. Talent will not; nothing is more common than unsuccessful men with talent. Genius will not; unrewarded genius is almost a proverb. Education will not; the world is full of educated derelicts. Persistence and determination alone are omnipotent. The slogan 'Press On' has solved and always will solve the problems of the human race." – Calvin Coolidge

Being persistent is an overwhelming determinate of success in virtually any endeavor. It is the only way you will be able to find out *how successful you can be at any given undertaking.*

Talent and other innate gifts do play *some* role in how good you eventually become. The most important thing is for you to understand that you will only realize *your* full potential by working persistently at a task.

In this course, you have no idea how successful you can be until you *do the work!!!*

This program is about realizing your unique potential. Understand that at the start, you have no idea how successful you can be.

In my experience, most people are stunned to find that they can accomplish a huge amount more than they believed possible. They had carried fixed mindset beliefs that limited what they were willing to attempt because *they assumed they would fail.*

Embrace the growth mindset. In the real world you never really know what you can do until you work at it!

Positive Energy

Taking on a new challenge will require the best effort you can muster. One of the most important conditions for putting out your best effort will be lots of positive energy.

The energy will come from yourself and your attitude, and from those around you

You begin every day with a "can do" attitude and get excited about your training and what you are going to accomplish. You feel the power of your own enthusiasm propelling you to make changes and do the things you know are needed.

Positive energy is contagious. When you dive into a task with positive enthusiasm, it energizes those around you to feel good and do their best.

Positive energy will lift you up and move you ahead. Negative energy will do just the opposite.

Negative energy feels like it sucks the air out of a room. Tasks that may have seemed a little difficult now become impossible.

Having a positive attitude can make hard work seem enjoyable. It helps you surge forward and embrace the next challenge.

A negative attitude can do just the opposite. It can stop you in your tracks before you even get started. Negativity hangs in the air like a bad smell and can undercut everything you try to do.

Being around negative people can drain your energy quickly. For them life appears to be a trudge from one bad experience to another. They find fault with everything. They will assure you that trying to get back in good condition is going to fail.

For negative people "nothing ever works", there is always "a reason (fill in the blank) will fail", or "it is pointless to try".

You should stay as far away from these people as possible. They will do nothing but suck energy out of you. They are the last people you want to be around when you are trying to do something difficult.

Hang out with people who are positive and enthusiastic, particularly about your desire to get back in good condition. Their positive energy will multiply your energy.

Take Action

If someone delays acting, the chances are that they won't do anything. Procrastination (or inaction) becomes the normal way of life.

Here is a prime example. According to surveys done by national polling firms, roughly 1/3 of the adults in the United States *claim* that they do vigorous exercise for at least 30 minutes three times a week.

Researchers at the University of Washington decided to check the validity of this claim by attaching sensors to people for a month. What they found was that while 33% of the population claimed to exercise three times a week, the number that actually did work out three times a week was a modest 6%.

In short, people believe they *should* work out, but the overwhelming majority don't.

Why?

I suspect that there are lot of reasons, and that the mix is different from one person to another. However, I think that there are some common issues that impact just about everyone to some degree.

Many have good intentions. But they avoid *acting.* The longer they put off taking action the less likely it is that they will ever DO something.

Then there is the opposite condition where some people are constantly "over-active".

Healthy High Achievement

One of the big issues that confront many people at age 50 and above is how to achieve some reasonable balance in their lives between work, family and taking care of themselves.

Typically, those of us who have been brought up to be high achievers find that we don't have nearly "enough time" to do all the things we believe are "critical". We are putting in 60+ hour weeks at work, not caring for our health as we should, and not doing what we want to with our families.

We are constantly on our laptops, phones, or tablets because we believe there is always something in our work that needs our immediate attention.

As much effort as we may put in to any given task, it never seems to be enough. The outcome could "always be better". There is always more to do.

You may be working your ass off and not getting much feeling of satisfaction from it.

Now, along comes this *exercise book!!* (The one in your hand). How it is possible to get in good shape with all the other things you "have to" do?

For openers, it can help to realize that there is this belief widely held among high achievers called "perfectionism" that makes it nearly impossible to ever be satisfied with anything one does.

Perfectionism is the completely fallacious idea that somehow it is possible to do many things "perfectly". Something not possible in the real world.

The quote from Vince Lombardi, one of the most famous of all "perfectionists", provides some insight. He said you can "always pursue perfection, you will never get there, but along the way discover excellence."

The bottom line is that you do the best you can given the constraints imposed by time and your energy. Doing the best you can in the time you have is the essence of what the late Admiral Rickover meant when he said, "All I want is the best you can do. I don't know of anyone anywhere who can do more than that."

Being a high achiever means that you may routinely place a lot of extreme expectations on yourself. It is likely that "doing a great job" is one of the ways you got a lot of your approval and recognition in your life. This approval may have come from parents, family, co-workers, etc. In short, you were "proving yourself".

It is possible that your being driven may still be a means of trying to prove yourself. If you recognize this, and drop the emotional overhead, you will probably do just as good a job, but feel some satisfaction in your accomplishment.

I realize that a short course on fitness may not solve all the problems about how you may deal with the challenges of being a high achiever. However, it can help point the way for you to begin feeling good about the remarkable things you accomplish.

Thoughts on "discipline"

OK...you are *committed* to getting back in shape. But, how do you get yourself to *do* what is necessary, particularly when you may not *want* to do something at a specific time.

The word "discipline" comes to mind. This means doing something you know you *should* even though your body may not *want to*. The *real* successes in life come from having the discipline to do something that may not be appealing at first.

You have exercised discipline in your life before, probably many times. If you built a successful career, the early work was not easy, and often not fun. If you mastered a difficult subject in school, you probably had to endure many hours of difficult study. If you learned to play a musical instrument, you had to do a lot of practice when you were a real novice.

Getting back in shape is no different. In the early going some parts of the experience may be difficult for you, and you will have to use *discipline* to keep on course.

The good news is that the longer you stick with an exercise program, the more it becomes enjoyable!

For now, you need to understand the forces that will be working on you in the first month, and how to combat them.

One big issue you may face is that during each day you won't always have the discipline resources you want to keep on course. You will almost always have more discipline and commitment early in the day as opposed to later.

Every day, you begin with a limited supply of "discipline units". If you think about these units as if they were cash, it is like having an allowance that will not quite cover everything you may require during the day.

Assume you charge off to work with a lot of enthusiasm, and immediately get stuck in traffic making you late for your first meeting. This is followed with another meeting run by a guy who thinks that you have all the time in the world to listen to his endless rambling. Five minutes of substance crammed into an hour-long presentation.

It takes a bunch of your discipline units not to strangle the guy.

You still have a 3 PM deadline, and all these people are burning up your time with drivel.

The phone rings and on the other end is a person with an unsolvable problem. It might be easily solved it they had bothered to read the e-mail you sent them three days ago.

More discipline units get spent when you are polite to the guy…(a client).

As you go through the day, your discipline units get spent on dealing with people and situations that make you want to move to Mars. By 5 PM you are flat out of discipline units for the day, and still must deal with dinner, drinks, and the workout you have not yet completed.

Well…forget the workout today…not enough time. The day has been sh*t, and you "deserve" a few drinks to unwind. Dinner is good…and then come the chocolate chip cookies for dessert. The discipline units are all spent, and the cookies win big time.

"Well…I'll do better tomorrow."

Give that one a resounding "maybe".

You must understand that the pressures to quit will always be the strongest later in the day when you have exhausted your supply of discipline units. Since this is the case, you want to try and schedule your training sessions early in the day.

Another element of discipline is that sticking with your eating program will be easiest early in the day and fade as you get toward bed time.

If you understand this, create situations where you avoid temptations late in the day. Knowing what you are dealing with, you can anticipate having to exercise discipline over your impulses when your resolve may be at its lowest ebb.

Daily Recommitment

Everyone, including you, who starts a reconditioning program begins with great enthusiasm. This is great, because that positive enthusiasm will help keep you on course.

Renew your positive energetic commitment *every day*. This will begin your day super charged with good energy. Keep your vision of what you want to achieve clearly in mind.

Begin every day by looking in the mirror and recommitting to building your body, eating properly, and living a fit lifestyle. Say the words aloud. Look yourself in the eyes when you say them. Make these intentions "real".   Make your vision real.

This is a great way to start the day…but the effect can wear off quickly if you don't understand that many forces around you will conspire to disrupt or undercut your commitment.

How do you stay on course when "life" is doing everything possible to subvert your best intentions?

Remind yourself that your fitness program is something that will grow and improve *every day.* Anything of value takes time and work to accomplish. This program is worthy of your time and effort over a long period of time.

Think of your fitness program as something you are *doing not just for yourself, but for everyone who cares about you.*

Your health and fitness are critically important to everyone around you. You can be someone who sets a great example for your family, is physically able to be there for them when needed, and successfully meets challenges when they arise.

This is not just about looking good for a week or two on vacation. It is about having a life that will impact everyone around you in a positive way.

You must also remind yourself that *you are "the boss" of what happens to you.* You and you alone decide to work out, and what to eat.

That is a lot different from someone who is constantly at the mercy of even the smallest life events.

You are *always in charge. Remember that and repeat it to yourself throughout the day.*

Do the workouts! Eat right every day. Commit to getting better every day!

As the Nike commercial used to say: "Just DO it!"

Your Daily Regimen

1. **Recommit to your vision, and to your exercise and nutrition program multiple times each day.** Commit out loud to yourself in front of the mirror every morning. You can also say it to yourself in the mid afternoon when your energy and discipline begins to fade. Say it to yourself at night as you go to bed. Your vision will power you along the path of progress.
2. **Adopt a Growth Mentality -** There is NO way to determine in advance what your actual potential is in any endeavor. You will only find out what your real potential is by working at becoming as good as you can be.
3. **Be positive and surround yourself with people who have positive energy.** There is nothing that will give your commitment more power than a positive and eager attitude. Embrace difficulty with enthusiasm, and charge ahead. Avoid people who are negative or exude negative energy.
4. **Remember that persistence is the ONLY way to succeed.** This applies whether you are doing physical training or trying to learn Physics. You must consistently <u>take action</u> and the desired results will come.
5. **What happened in the past does not determine what happens now –** Bad past experiences or frustrations should remain in the past and not be an anchor on your present work. Push through your fear to the triumph! You will feel the huge satisfaction that comes from doing something that is difficult.

Month
2

"It takes as much time to be mediocre as it does to be successful...."

- Ryan Lee

"Always pursue perfection. You will never get there, but along the way you will discover excellence..."

-Vince Lombardi

Month 2

The quest continues

Renew your vision

Congratulations! You have successfully completed a month of reconditioning training. You have made a great start on getting back into the type of shape you desire. You are not only stronger and more resilient, you probably notice that you look better than when you started.

You should have your vision of who you want to become firmly in mind. You should continue to re-affirm your vision every day.

You will notice that you are becoming increasingly like your vision. You will have more muscle than you had when you started, and perhaps you have lost a few inches on your waist line.

You are probably thinking of yourself as becoming a "fit person". This means that your workouts, eating, and mindset are aligning to help you become this person. You don't have to fight to resist junk food. Ignoring it seems more natural.

In short, you are gradually becoming the person in your vision.

In month 2 of this program you will be doing more demanding exercises, becoming more focused and disciplined in your nutrition, and using your mind to help you work toward mastering the skills of fitness.

Month 2

Weight training: Building muscular endurance

In this month your training will focus on building more muscular endurance. This means raising your own personal conditioning baseline.

In the first phase of this program you got your body used to training with weights again and began reactivating the neural pathways that will be critical to building up your strength and athleticism.

In Month 2 of the program we devote primary attention to building up endurance, both muscular and cardiovascular. We will also focus on improving your balance, coordination, and general athleticism.

One of the main ways we do this is to use free weights (dumbbells and barbells). When you must control a weight in each hand, your stabilizer muscles are activated to the max. As I noted earlier, if you use a machine to do a lift, you get zero benefit for your athletic coordination.

In this phase of training you will be using weights that are relatively light for you. As you are reconditioning, you will be rebuilding;

- Muscle density
- Strength in a full range of motion
- Strength and resilience in connective tissues
- Mobility in joints
- Better muscular coordination
- Enhanced cardiovascular endurance

Weight training routine in Month 2 will be done as follows:

- Do all exercises for **3 sets of 8-10 repetitions**
- Begin using weights that you can do relatively easily for 6-7 reps
- Never exceed 80% effort on any rep
- Increase the weight 5 lbs. when you can do 10 reps and drop back to doing 8 reps
- Move briskly; no more than 60-90 seconds between sets of any exercise
- Take no more than 2 minutes between exercises

Aerobic training in Month 2 will be:

- Low intensity aerobics for 10-15 minutes after the weight workout
- Train 3 days per week
- If you desire, you can alternate weight training days and aerobic training days

Remember, low intensity aerobics are very important in rebuilding your strength and fitness. The purpose is to begin rebuilding your cardiovascular system (heart, lungs, arteries, veins, and capillaries). If you have been inactive for some time, your cardio system will need gradual rehabilitation.

Month 2 will be a little more challenging than the first month.

Month 2

Exercises

1. Overhead barbell press (3 sets x 8 reps)
2. Bench press (3 x 8)
3. Bent over rowing (3 x 8)
4. Barbell curl (3 x 8)
5. Triceps press (3 x 8)
6. Goblet squat (3 x 8)
7. Deadlift (3 x 8)
8. Kettlebell/dumbbell swing (3 x 8)
9. Leg raises (3 sets – work up to 10-15 reps)

Month 2: Weight Training Program

Critical Point: Lifting with Excellent Technique

Most fitness trainees devote minimal attention to proper performance of various lifts. This results in their getting sub-optimal results from their training and getting injured regularly. It is not widely understood that poor technique is a common cause of routine gym injuries.

Without excellent technique, you will never be able to get anywhere near your full potential and minimize your chance for injury. With poor technique, you also get less benefit from each exercise than if you did it right.

As you want to get back in good condition, and not have your progress slowed or stopped by injuries, I'll devote a lot of attention to proper lifting technique.

I include detailed descriptions of how to do each lift. Pay careful attention to these instructions and work to insure you have the best technique possible every time you lift a weight

Achieving perfect lifting technique is something that cannot be done overnight. You should begin training with the goal of perfecting your lifting technique over time. This is no easy task, but persistence is the key to success.

---

1. Overhead barbell press

Most of the lifts will be done standing on your feet. As I harp on continually, this is essential for building your balance, coordination, and strength.

In the first month you did the two-hand dumbbell press. In Month 2 you will be introduced to one of the greatest weightlifting movements of all time: the overhead barbell press.

Begin by selecting a weight that you can lift relatively easily for seven of the eight reps in the set. You may have to experiment to find the weight that is works best for you.

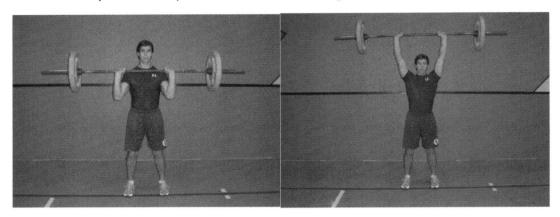

Standing Overhead Barbell Press – Starting position and "lock out" position

Start with the barbell the floor. Stand with your feet slightly wider than shoulder width, with your toes aligned. Bend over and pick the weight off the floor and bring it up to your right shoulders in one motion. This movement is called the "clean". It is a great conditioning exercise that is part of advanced training.

When the bar is at your shoulders, tighten your entire body from the tips of your toes to the top of your head. Being completely tight will help you *recruit* power from every muscle as you do the lift.

Take a deep breath and hold it. Tense your body and drive the barbell overhead in one smooth motion. Push the barbell just past your nose and once it clears your head, push it slightly back so that you are driving it to arm's length over the center of your head.

Your knees should be rigid and not bend as you push the bar upward. You should not give the weight any upward momentum by flexing your knees and jerking. The power should come entirely from your arms, shoulders, and tightly flexed body.

You should squeeze the bar as you press. This will help activate all the muscles in your arm, shoulder, back, and legs. Keep your abs tight. You should feel the tension of the pressing movement in your abs.

Your elbows should be straight and not flexed when you finish the press to the "lock out" position. Release your breath and lower the weight to your shoulders to do another rep. When the bar is back at your shoulders again, take another breath and do the next rep.

When you have done the required number of repetitions, return the bar to the floor, and recover before you do the next set.

In most of the lifts in this course, you will be *recruiting* all the muscle power you can from everywhere in your body. It is exactly the opposite of *isolation* which emphasizes using a few muscles to do a lift and kills any chance you have to build serious strength.

When doing the overhead press, you should begin with the barbell on the floor. *Never take it off a squat rack.* There are multiple reasons for this. The biggest is that lifting off the floor builds coordination, athleticism, and strength. It also primes your body to put out serious force when you are ready to press. Another reason is that taking the bar off a squat rack makes you look totally lame.

2. Bench Press

The bench press is one of the most popular lifts in the world. It is one of the lifts used in competitive powerlifting along with the deadlift and squat.

These three lifts form the core of the programs I use to build long term strength and fitness. However, it takes time to develop the skill needed to get maximum benefit from them. So, I only introduce them in this reconditioning course. Mastering them comes later.

It is a good idea for you *not* to attempt any heavy bench presses until you have finished Month 3 of this course. At this point, you are still in the early stages of your reconditioning, and doing heavy lifts is counterproductive. You also run the risk of injury.

Good bench-pressing technique begins by positioning yourself correctly on the bench. The picture below shows what your alignment should be.

Your shoulders and buttocks should be in contact with the bench. You should have a slight arch in your lower back. Your feet should be positioned so that your toes are behind the knees. Your entire body should be tight enough so that if a forklift picked you up off the bench, you would be frozen in position. You must keep this tightness throughout the entire set.

Keeping your whole body tight during the bench press is essential if you want to develop a powerful press and get full benefit from your training. If you relax any part of your body during this lift it is like having a leak in a hydraulic system. All the pressure in the system dissipates.

The lift begins with the bar at arm's length over your face, as shown in the picture. Take a deep breath and hold it. Push your shoulders down toward your toes.

Lower the bar slowly to a point _at the bottom of your rib cage_. The bar should touch your solar plexus. It should _not_ touch farther up your chest around the nipples.

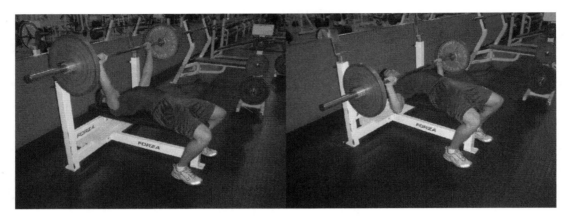

Starting position   Bar on chest ready for upward press

If you land the bar high on the chest the lift is being done entirely by the small muscles in your frontal deltoids and triceps. In short, you can generate minimal power with that technique. Landing the bar lower on your chest allows you to involve the lats and your pectoral muscles.

Keep your butt firmly on the bench. Every muscle in your body should be tight when the bar is on your chest. If you relax, the weight will squash you like a ripe grape.

As you push on the bar to drive it upward, it should travel in an arc back up to the position you started where the bar was over your face. You should be able to feel the "groove" where you are able to exert maximum power and have maximum stability.

When the bar is roughly ¾ of the way back to the starting position, you release your breath. You will have to inhale (and hold) your breath again at the start of the next repetition.

Stand up between sets. Do not recline on the bench.

3. Bent over rowing

This is a great exercise for the whole back, especially the lats. It will also work your arms and abdominal muscles.

Begin with the barbell on the floor. Bend over at the waist and grasp the barbell with a grip slightly wider than shoulder width.

Tense your abdominal muscles, tighten your legs, back and hips. Push your shoulders down toward your waist, tighten your grip on the barbell. Take a deep breath and hold it.

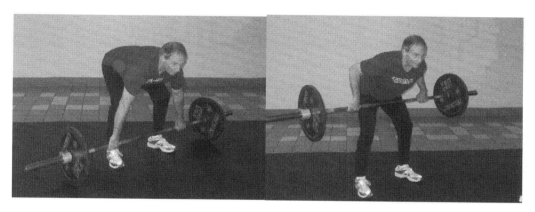

Bent over rowing: start

Bent over rowing: top position

Pull the barbell upward to your *waist*. When you touch your waist, gradually lower the weight back to the floor and exhale.

4. Barbell Curl

Everyone seems to love having good looking biceps. For this reason, curls are a very popular exercise. Last month you did curls with dumbbells, this month with a barbell.

There are a lot of functional reasons for having strong biceps, not the least of which is that they are involved in any lifting movement you do.

Load the barbell with the weight you intend to use, then grasp it with palms facing outward and stand erect. When you are ready to start the curl, your arms should be hanging straight down beside you.

Begin by taking a deep breath and holding it. Your entire body should be tense before you begin to move the weight. Bring the barbell to your shoulders with your palms facing up. Keep your elbows against your sides. When the bar reaches your shoulders, your palms should be facing in toward your body.

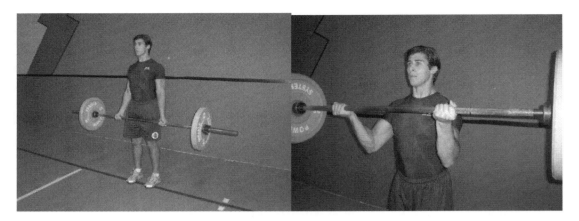

Barbell curl: starting position   Halfway to the shoulders

It is important that you fully extend each arm at the start of each curl. In reconditioning, one of the things you will be training is developing strength in a full range of motion. Thus, you do not want to "cheat" by starting a curl with a slightly bent arm.

Keep very strict form even though it will mean that you do not use a very big weight.

Keep an erect posture throughout the entire exercise, and do NOT use any body movement that would allow you to use a bigger weight.

5. Triceps Press

The companion exercise to the curl is the triceps press. This works the muscles on the back of the arm.

The triceps is essential to every pushing or pressing movement you do. The dumbbell movement here is intended to enhance strength in the full range of motion for the triceps.

Begin by holding one end of a dumbbell in both hands. Push the dumbbell overhead to arm's length, still holding one end in both hands.

Take a deep breath and slowly lower the weight behind your head. Try to keep your elbows pointed directly upward.

Lower the weight behind your head as far as you can go without experiencing pain. Keeping the elbows pointed upward, use your triceps to push the weight back to a point where it is directly overhead.

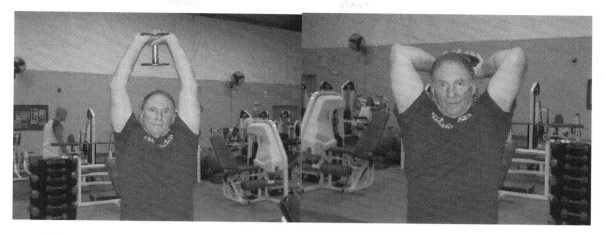

Triceps press: starting position   Triceps press: lower position

As in the curl, strict form is more important than the amount of weight you use. The purpose of this phase of training is getting your full range of motion restored.

6. Kettlebell/Dumbbell Goblet Squat

The squat is the king of body strength exercises and should be a mainstay in any conditioning program.

In reconditioning it is particularly important that you focus on restoring your full range of motion. Most people who reach age 50 will have lost a lot of flexibility and strength in squatting motions.

If you had problems with your knees or back when doing the unweighted squat, you should continue to work without weights until you can easily perform squats.

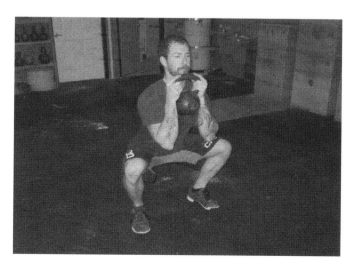

Kettlebell squat (aka. "goblet" squat)

Leg press or leg extension machines are NOT a proxy for doing free standing squats. Machine lifts will rob you of your ability to balance and control weights in space. In short, the machine will suck all the athletic performance out of any lift.

Begin standing upright with your feet slightly wider than shoulder width. You will be holding a kettlebell (or dumbbell) just below your chin. Hold the kettlebell by each side of the handle or hold a dumbbell by one end.

Take a deep breath and hold it. Push your hips back and descend into a full squat. When you have reached full squat depth, immediately come back to a standing position. Exhale when you are about ¾ of the way back to the starting position.

You should keep an upright posture throughout the lift. If you roll forward, you will place a lot of strain on your back, and have difficulty keeping your balance.

This exercise will help restore your full range of motion, and when you use proper form, build a powerful abdominal core.

As in other exercises in the restoration program, you are aiming at building good range of motion and good muscle endurance, not going for heavy weights and all you can lift.

7. Deadlift

The deadlift is one of the training movements that can build extraordinary body strength. It is perhaps *the* exercise that will prevent you from getting a "bad back" as you age.

The lift appears simple if you have never done it. In reality it is more complicated than you might think. Good technique is essential if you are going to get the benefit from this lift,

You will again be aiming at establishing a full range of motion and building muscular endurance. Thus, heavy weights are to be avoided. Going heavy too early, even if the lift seems easy, is a bad idea.

Initially, you should work on "good" technique in your deadlift. As you progress, it will be critical that you *perfect* your lifting technique. At this stage of your training learning basic form.

Begin with the barbell on the floor in front of you. Set up with your feet about 12 inches apart (30 cm). Your shins should be touching the bar.

Take a deep breath and hold it while you go down and grasp the bar. The air in your lungs will compress and help create a lot of tension in your body when you go into position to pull the weight.

Next, tighten your entire body. That is tense every muscle everywhere. This is a "whole body" lift and you need every muscle to be tight if you are going to put out full power.

Keeping your butt down and your back flat, lower your hips down until you can grasp the bar with both hands.

At no time should you round your back. It must always be flat (the "power pulling" position) during the lift.

Your head should be held erect, and you should fix your eyes on a spot on the wall in front of you. Keep your eyes on that spot throughout the pull.

Keeping your entire body tense, stand erect with the weight.

When you pull the weight off the floor, you should keep your butt down and your back completely flat. NEVER allow your shoulders to "roll over" so your back is rounded.

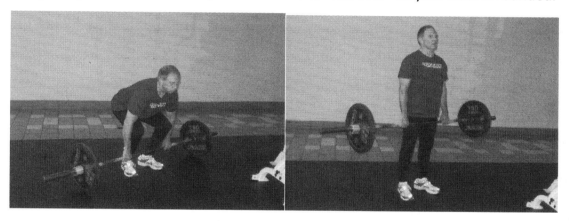

Deadlift – Starting position   Deadlift – finishing position

You should feel tension in your abdominal muscles when you pull. This will tell you that your body alignment is correct. If you feel stress in your lower back, either your butt and hips are too high.

When you have come to a full standing position, release your breath, then slowly lower the weight back to the floor.

DO NOT jerk the weight off the floor or try to move quickly. Until your body is fully adapted to performing the deadlift, sudden movements or jerking the weight are very likely to cause injuries.

In this phase of your re-conditioning, you can simply "touch" the weight on the floor and stand erect again. Later you will have the weight to come to a full stop on the floor between reps.

I cannot stress enough that in re-conditioning you will be working to build your muscular endurance and learn good technique. Forget heavy weights for now. You will be able to get more aggressive with heavier weights later. For now, train smart.

You should NOT wear a lifting belt during this (or any other) re-conditioning exercise. The lifting belt is only for doing very heavy lifting.

The purpose of re-conditioning is to build up your body to do a variety of complex movements. Wearing support gear, such as belts, wraps, or gloves, weakens you. This is because you become dependent on the equipment to carry the load, not your muscles.

8. Kettlebell/Dumbbell Swing

The swing is an exercise that has a *huge* positive impact on your overall conditioning. Don't be deceived by the relative simplicity of the movement. The swing enhances your muscular endurance, balance, coordination, aerobic capacity, and whole-body muscularity.

The swing is also a dynamite fat burner.

It is worth mentioning that there are two different exercises called "the swing". They accomplish different things, but for some reason have the same name. The version I'll show you here is the "Hard Style" or "Russian" swing. I use this extensively in my own training.

(The other version of the swing is taught in Cross-Fit and some other gyms. In that exercise, you lift the weight overhead).

In the "Hard Style" version of the swing, you will only lift the weight to a point where your arms are parallel to the floor.

You should begin swing training with light weights. It is important that you can do the three sets of eight reps feeling refreshed rather than "toasted".

Start by holding a kettlebell or dumbbell with both hands in front of you. Your feet should be slightly wider than shoulder width apart.

Take a deep breath and hold it. Then sit back as if you were going to sit in a chair and swing the weight back between your legs as if you were hiking a football.

Keep your back flat, with hips lower than your shoulders. Your head should be up, but not exaggerated. Look straight ahead.

When the weight is behind you, forcefully drive it forward and up using your hips and abdominal muscles. Don't pull with your arms at all. They are merely "ropes" holding the weight for you in this exercise.

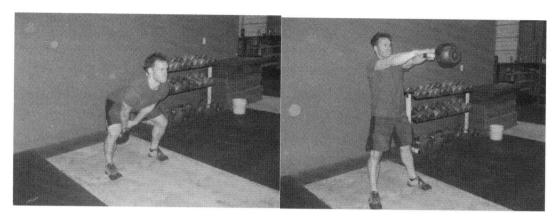

Swing – Bottom position ("hike")   Swing – Top position - arms parallel to floor

The drive from the "hike" position should be done by your hamstrings, glutes and abdominal muscles. This comes from quickly straightening your legs while driving your hips forward. At the same time, flex your glutes.

To drive to the finish position, you should lean back slightly, pinch your glutes together and flex your abs.

The final drive should bring the weight to a point where your arms are parallel to the floor.

For a split second the weight will go motionless or "float" when your arms are parallel. At that point quickly release your breath. You will quickly inhale again as the weight descends.

You want to have a full breath with tight abdominals when you are ready to drive the weight upward again.

Allow the weight to swing back between your legs and then drive it upward again. Each upward swing is a repetition.

DO NOT use your arms in any way to propel the weight. Think of your arms merely as "ropes" that hold the weight you are driving up using your hip drive and abdominal muscles to move.

9. Leg Raise

Begin lying on your back on the floor. Place your hands at your sides. Take a deep breath and hold it. Keeping your legs straight, raise your feet off the floor until your legs are elevated to a 45-degree angle.

Lower your legs back to the starting position under full control. Set your feet gently back on the floor and release your breath.

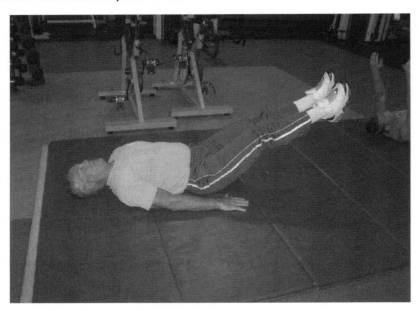

Leg Raise

If this exercise is too difficult with straight legs, bend your knees slightly so that you can do the required number of reps.

Don't bounce your feet off the floor when you are doing reps. Start each repetition from a dead stop.

Month 2 Aerobic Training

Following your weight workout, do 10-15 minutes of the aerobic training mode of your choice. You should be able to *increase the pace or tempo* a bit over that you used in Month 1. However, remember the purpose of these reconditioning programs is to get you ready to do more aggressive workouts. So, remember, "train...don't strain".

This month you should gradually increase the total time you spend doing low intensity aerobic training. The purpose will be to build up your baseline capacity so that next month you can begin doing more demanding "interval" training.

Remember that the purpose of aerobic training is to build up the capacity of your heart, lungs, and circulation system. If you have been sedentary for a long time your entire cardiovascular system will have deteriorated from what it was in your youth.

It is possible to rebuild extraordinary cardio fitness, but it must be done gradually. You can build incredible capacity, but it takes time.

If you are overweight it is particularly important that you *gradually* retrain your body to deal with the stresses of cardio training. You really don't want to get an injury to a tendon or joint during your reconditioning.

You must also remember that doing a lot of cardio training will not help you much for losing fat. If you are overweight, you won't be able to run fast enough or long enough to make much of a dent in your fat stores. Fat loss will come from proper eating and the cumulative effect of regular training.

Month 2: Nutrition

Keep doing what you learned to do in Month 1

You made a lot of important progress in the first month. Kicking the sugar habit is huge for many people. Being aware of what you're eating and making conscious choices to eat something or not eat something is a major accomplishment.

In the second month, we will build on the first month and move ahead even more.

Now we begin to explore choices that will be best for your long-term welfare.

Dieting vs Fit Lifestyle

If you are going to enjoy a good experience getting back in shape, it is essential that you establish routine eating patterns that support a fit body. As I noted earlier, this means you will be building a "fit lifestyle", not "going on a diet".

There is a big difference between the two.

Dieters seem to be on a quest that never ends. At least it rarely ends with any continuing success.

Dieting seems to be one of those activities where people are either "on" or "off". When they are "on" a diet, life with food seems to be characterized by the "Four D's". That is: deprivation, discipline, depression, and despair.

People "on" a diet are dealing with a sentence imposed from outside their personal orbit. Whatever else is happening in their life, the dieters can bitch that they are "not allowed" to eat certain things. This carping is often coupled with regular reminders to anyone listening that the dieter is virtuous and humble. They deserve many props for saving the planet from excess ass fat.

When someone is "off" a diet, life with food is characterized by the acronym GLEE. That is: Gluttony, License, Euphoria and Excess.

Whatever cosmic power that was keeping them "on" the diet, has vanished. Lacking the restraints imposed by the diet gods, almost anything goes. Forget spoonful's, bring on the shovels!

It is almost a cliché that people who diet and lose weight will quickly put the pounds back on once they reach their "goal". If they "drop 50", they will put it all back on within a year and add some extra.

Once the "weight loss" goal has been reached, that is the signal to forget the dog days of the 4D's and embrace "GLEE".

At that point, the devotees of "diet sport" will begin another program of sacrifice to reduce their personal bulk.   This is the infamous "diet yo-yo".

Eating as part of a fit lifestyle is quite a different experience.

Eating is one of many things that are done purposefully and by a conscious choice. The choice begins with how you want to live your life. One of the first choices is whether you want to be constantly at war with your body. This is the difference between wanting to "eat to live", or "live to eat".

Anyone on the GLEE program can say they *purposefully* selected the bag of chocolate chip cookies and *chose* to eat the whole thing. They might also argue that the cookies were necessary to live.

For people "at war" with their bodies this type of eating is not about *needing* to eat, but rather about using food (or drink) as gratification for something else.   For these folks eating offers temporary comfort. Food becomes a short-lived substitute for some unmet "need".

The big problem is that since the "need" these people are trying to fix is most likely not related to food, they can never eat enough.

Moral of the story is that you need to be clear about what you are eating and why. Eating as a substitute for something else will undercut any chance you have for becoming fit.

Fit Lifestyle Eating

A big part of eating as part of a fit lifestyle is getting your head on straight. It is about "eating to live" as opposed to "living to eat".

Your meals are to support a fit body, not meet some "other" type of need. You eat when you *need* food, not when some insecurity is triggered.

If you are not hungry, you don't eat. There is no drama around this.

You decide what to eat and when. You are not on some externally imposed "diet" to regulate your behavior.

After a while, you will find that eating this way becomes your "new normal" pattern. It may take some discipline to get into this pattern. Once established it should take minimal discipline to stick to it.

Getting to the place where your habitual eating pattern conforms to a fit lifestyle may take some time to accomplish. For some people it will only take a few weeks. Others will have to work at this longer.

The important thing is that it be part of your vision of yourself and how you want to be in the long term.

Eat Like the Person you want to become

Last month I said that if you want to be a 175-pound athlete instead of a 225-pound blob, eat like the athlete, and that is what you will gradually become.

That guidance still holds true. But, a month in to this program you need to evaluate the impact of the changes you made to your eating habits last month. Hopefully, you have seen some significant positive changes.

This month take a hard look at the total volume of food you are eating. If you are eating good food, but have not lost a lot of fat, you may have to reduce the quantity of food you eat.

It is always a good idea to look for "stealth" calories or previously unseen sources of grazing.

I probably don't need to tell you that beer and other alcohol drinks are loaded with calories. Just because you don't eat it with a fork doesn't mean that it doesn't count as part of your caloric food intake.

The same goes for the morning coffee stop. You can take on 1000 calories with a mocha latte and a "bran" muffin. Black coffee is zero calories. Coffee with 3 sugar packets is about 60 calories.

Building more good habits

This month you will continue to build more good habits that will be part of your fit lifestyle. The more you practice doing the right things, the easier it will be to sustain them in the long term.

Eating fresh produce

Every sports nutrition program I know of extolls the value of eating fresh produce. Most weight loss programs encourage you to eat as many veggies as possible.

If you want to eat organic vegetables, that is fine. The nutrition content of non-organic vegetables is virtually the same as organic (source: Harvard Medical School). The main thing is to eat FRESH veggies.

The obvious caveat to this is that there are a variety of products that masquerade as vegetables that are little more than fat bombs. I'm referring to French fries, potato chips, corn chips, hash browns, etc.

You should build your veggie eating around having lots of different vivid colors. Examples: the dark greens of broccoli, green beans, and spinach; the vivid colors of peppers; the array of green shades in spring greens, etc.

If you don't currently eat a lot of fresh veggies, you should begin eating them every day.

You will have to try different vegetables and combinations to see what you like. Enjoy grazing.

Adequate protein

When you train for strength, your training tears down muscle in workouts, and your recovery period is when the muscle (and other tissues) re-build and get stronger. This is the basic principle of training. The body responds to physical stresses by building muscle and aerobic capacity.

To optimize recovery, you should insure that you have adequate daily protein intake. This will vary from person to person, but as a rule, you should ingest a minimum of 1 gram of protein for every 4 pounds (2 kilos) of lean bodyweight.

I am aware that there are numerous advertisements and promotions that suggest you should gobble protein (usually the vendors supplement) at staggering rates. I'll offer two thoughts:

1) You are getting *back into condition* and taking excessive amounts of protein, particularly supplements, won't help you. The extra calories can become fat
2) In re-conditioning, it is important that you reestablish eating habits that provide your nutrition from *food*.

Depending on your preferred diet, you should insure that you are eating adequate protein. The

You should estimate your protein needs based on the body weight you *want to achieve.*

Avoiding unplanned pig-outs

I'm not suggesting that you need to become a monk or an anti-social wedge-ass, but there are some routine social situations that can blast away some of your best intentions and hard work.

Topping the list is any version of "going out for a few drinks". Alcoholic drinks have a lot of calories of the kind that are quickly converted to "table muscle". You should be aware of how much you drink, because you can eat like a spartan rabbit all day, and then blow it by downing a pizza and washing it down with a six-pack.

Another problem with the going out for drinks scenario is that after a few "pops", your resistance to eating a bunch of chips, peanuts or other bar food may be significantly reduced.

I don't need to go on about different opportunities to blow your eating program. I'll only offer the following observation from my own experience.

You don't have to skip social invitations or miss parties because you are "on a program". You exercise restraint about what you eat and how much you drink. No one cares if you drink 2 beers or 10. You control what goes in your mouth and enjoy the company of your friends.

It is also worth noting that if you choose not to drink alcohol, it is not necessary to announce it to your companions. I speak from the experience of being a non-drinker.

I don't skip parties, I accept social invitations, and all my adult family members drink alcohol. The bottom line is that no one cares whether you drink alcohol or not. The only time they are likely to notice is when someone needs to be a designated driver. At that point, the non-drinker temporarily assumes the status of a "first round draft choice".

Do calories count?

There has been a lot of discussion of late about the importance of counting calories if you want to lose fat. My bottom line on the role of calories in fat loss, is that while calories may not be the *only* thing that impacts obesity, it definitely is a factor.

You should develop a *clear sense* of how much _you_ can eat and lose fat. Remember, each of us is somewhat unique.

I'll give a quick story to show what I mean. The wife of one of my friends is about 5' 1" tall and weighs about 100 pounds. She eats like an NFL linebacker….and never gains an ounce. One of my weightlifter pals is about 6' tall, weighs about 205 lbs and quickly puts on fat if he eats more than one full meal and a snack.

You need to find out *how your unique metabolism works.* This is the only way you will ever be able to optimize your own eating. Experimenting is the only way you can find what is going to be valid for you.

As already noted, each of us has a different metabolism rate. Factors that impact the differences include:

- age (older people usually have lower basic metabolism rates than younger people)
- size (bigger people usually have higher base metabolic rates than small people)
- present physical condition (well-conditioned people burn fewer calories per unit of work than poorly conditioned people)
- unique metabolic rate (some people have the metabolism of a hummingbird, others the metabolism of a tree sloth)

As a rule, older people need fewer calories to maintain body functions than younger ones. A few years ago, the general rule was that people needed 1% fewer calories for each year after age 30.

This means that at age 50 the "average" person would need 20% fewer calories every day than they did at age 30.

While this is not a hard and fast rule, it appears to be generally true and one that all of us have to consider as we age.

Another factor that is generally overlooked is that well-conditioned people burn fewer calories per unit of work than people who are in lousy shape.

I'll use an example from running as it is easy to explain.

Runner's World magazine used to publish a table showing how many calories an "average" runner would burn for each mile they ran. The variables were:

- Running speed – running faster requires more calories than slower
- Runners body weight – bigger runners burn more than smaller

The authors noted that as runners got in better shape, the number of calories needed per mile would drop because their bodies got more efficient. As oxygen uptake improves, so does the efficiency of all the runner's muscles.

Think for a minute about the running speed variable. Running at a 5:30 minute per mile pace is much more demanding than running at an 8:00 minute per mile pace. If you were in a zero-gravity environment this would not be true. On earth, we must overcome gravity, and inertia.

The point is that as you get in better condition, you will be using fewer calories to do the same amount of work.

Over time you may have to adjust your calorie intake as you get in better shape. Calorie intake will always be a moving target.

Month 2: Motivation and Mindset

Fit Lifestyle

By now you have been practicing a fit "lifestyle" for 30 days. Part of this lifestyle is the fundamental principal that you *choose* to do certain things or choose NOT to do other things.

- Workout on a regular schedule
- You eat like a fit person
- You have a growth and learning mindset

Doing your training is now a "regular" thing you do without any drama or trying to decide if you will work out today or not.

You choose what you eat and just as important, choose what NOT to eat.

Your mindset is that you are growing your skills toward mastering what you need to do to live the fit lifestyle.

You are conscious about making these choices.

As you drive into the second month of this program, it should be useful to look at potential pitfalls that may occur.

Ways to fail and keep failing

There are at least four major ways to fail when starting a fitness program:

- Finding excuses to quit
- Blaming failures or frustrations on others
- Expecting things to be "easy"
- Being overly self-critical

Looking for ways to quit is one of the most common impulses that confront someone starting a fitness program. Among the more common are:

- Fitness really is NOT that important
- I deserve a break from hard work
- My schedule is way too busy to fit this in
- I can do this next month...next year, etc.
- I'm in good shape for someone my age

The common theme in all these specific "reasons" for quitting is that the person does not want to continue the program. They need a legitimate sounding "reason" to justify quitting. So, any of the excuses above can sound reasonable enough for them to convince themselves, and perhaps others, that they are completely justified in blowing off a fitness program.

Deep down they know this is rubbish. However, the excuses offered can cover up the real reason they quit. The program seems too hard.

Another common set of excuses for quitting center around finding ways to blame others for problems that arise. Here are some common excuses:

- My failure is due to someone else screwing up
- It is not *really* a failure, it is normal for anyone to do this
- I can't be expected to succeed because of (fill in the blank)
- Whoever calls this a failure never had to do anything this difficult.

Then there is the person who deals with difficulty by becoming overly critical of themselves:

This is where instead of saying "I made a mistake", the person says (to themselves) something like "I am an idiot, etc." They see themselves as a "flawed person", not someone who made an error.

This approach virtually guarantees that no learning will occur. Any chance for improvement will be lost in a blizzard of self-criticism.

But, let's get back to getting physically fit and powerful over age 50.

For you to get into good condition, assume you will need to do a hell of a lot of work over weeks and months. Sometimes it will be frustrating or discouraging...or both.

That's the way it is. Developing proficiency means working through the steps needed to build skill, learning from mistakes, and commitment to constantly getting better.

Growing toward proficiency: Fit by Choice

You have embarked on a reconditioning program because it is vitally important to you and everyone you care about. You have successfully made it through the first month of training and have some solid results to celebrate.

The next stage of your revitalization will offer more challenges, and even greater rewards.

Your daily affirmations helped you stay on track during the first month. They are a daily recommitment to doing this training.

Now in your second month of working out, you can add another line to your daily look in the mirror.

This is one of the most powerful truths about physical training and the impact is has on you and your life. It comes from the great kettlebell master Pavel.

"When you live hard, life is easy. When you live easy, life is *hard!*"

The essence of this statement is that if a person takes the path of tough conditioning and disciplined eating, daily life goes on without concern for physical limitations, and has the enormous reward of feeling strong and healthy 24/7/365.

On the other hand, if a person chooses to live a life of physical ease, life becomes a horror show of chronic medical problems and physical frailty. Even easy physical tasks become difficult. Taking lots of prescription medications to maintain normal physical functions becomes necessary.

Living "easy" extracts a terrible price physically as well as mentally an emotionally.

The process of developing proficiency

Here is a simple but powerful way to think about the process of learning and developing proficiency. There are four distinct stages of learning that apply whether you are trying to learn organic chemistry or develop a fit body over age 50:

- Unconscious incompetence
- Conscious incompetence
- Conscious competence
- Unconscious competence

Everyone begins at the stage of unconscious incompetence. Literally, we "don't know what we don't know".

This is where most people are at the beginning of a fitness program. They don't really have a clue, but don't know that.

If they can persist through the first few sessions, they will begin to understand where their problems are. This is where diagnosis of specific problems that came up during the workout will be a huge help in identifying and specifying what needs work.

Doing the needed work will gradually get one to the point where they are consciously competent. This happens over time.

Eventually, a person can arrive at the point where they are unconsciously competent in *some* of the areas where they are working.

For example, most people are unconsciously competent doing something simple like driving a car. Such simple activities in life are the exception rather than the rule.

Most athletic (and intellectual) activities require continual feedback and correction. To master something requires prolonged commitment to working, testing and feedback.

If you don't believe this, why does no one's golf swing stay perfect after they do it right one time?

Increasing your chances for success

You are probably sick of hearing me say that when people first join a gym, or start working out, 90% will quit within three weeks.

Nine out of ten people who begin a quest for health and fitness *will completely abandon their program within three weeks of starting!!!!*

Why?

I believe one big reason is that *new trainees are not prepared to deal with the failures, fears, and frustrations they encounter.* They went into training *hoping* it would be relatively easy.

Here are a few examples of what I mean by this.

- Venturing into a gym is like visiting an alien planet for most new trainees. "Everyone else" seems to know what they are doing, and the new person has no clue.
- On top of feeling out of place, the various "exercises" make new people feel awkward if not downright clumsy. It is basically like being the new sophomore in a strange high school.
- The day following the "workout", the new trainee may have pain in places that had never hurt before.
- Getting to the gym for a second session may seem *very* inconvenient. There will be about 92 other activities that seem to have a higher priority than paying for being humbled, hurt, and embarrassed.

If you have been training in the relatively recent past, the shock and surprise may not be as great as if you are going into training for the first time.

If the new trainee manages to get through the first week on enthusiasm, by the second week the "glow" has begun to wear off. Nothing miraculous is going to happen overnight. Getting fit is going to be a *lot* of work.

The glitzy promotions about all the fun you are going to have, and how you will have a beach- ready body seem like promises from a politician.

The reality is that accomplishing anything worthwhile takes a lot of work. It also involves overcoming all kinds of frustration, failure, stress, self-doubt, and some other unpleasant experiences.

If you are over age 50, and "starting back" on the road to getting fit, it is essential that you *clearly understand* that you will experience failures along the way. ***Whether you succeed in achieving what you want will depend on how you respond to the failures you experience.***

Getting back in shape will be *extremely rewarding.* However, it will not be a stress-free walk in the park.

Embrace the difficulty. Nothing worth anything is accomplished without a lot of hard work and experiencing failure multiple times.

Learning from failures

Given that failures and frustrations will be part of any attempt to master something new, I'll offer you some tools for constructively dealing with these difficulties.

- **Every failure gives a lesson on something you need to learn**
- **Persistence is the most important thing in success**
- **Mastering anything involves failing several times**

Let's start with the idea that you *learn from your failures.*

Every *successful* athlete, business leader, scientist, writer, or anyone else learns from their mistakes or failures. The legendary Tom Watson who started the IBM Corporation once said basically that you never learn anything from success. The only time you learn is when you fail.

Michael Jordan, who became one of the greatest basketball players of all time, was cut from his high school basketball team (as a sophomore). He turned that around with hard work.

Once he got to the NBA, Jordan continued to learn from mistakes and grow as a player. Jordan once said "it took me seven years in the NBA to become Michael Jordan..." In those seven years, he took 56 "game winning" shots...and missed. To turn this around, he worked harder than any player in the history of the pro game.

Jordan is a stellar example of someone who made the most out of his talent by working hard and learning from his mistakes.

How do you "learn" from mistakes?

The first thing to do is be systematic about trying to learn. That is have a regular process that you use to figure out what went wrong and what you can do about it.

The process goes like this:

1. What happened (in detail)
2. Why do I think it happened as it did?
3. What do I intend to do about it next time?
4. Do I need a plan to work on this problem?

Diagnose the problem and look for potential solutions. Select solutions and try them out. Consciously look for ways to improve your performance.

The Monthly Review: A Methodology for Learning

There is a methodology you can use to benefit from the mistakes you make. This is known in the military as the "monthly review". This is your assessment of how you are doing, and what is going right, what is not up to par, and what you need to do.

This is the task of looking at what went wrong and why. It is not always pleasant. It can be downright unpleasant.

Begin by understanding that you "paid a price" for the experience you were just given. Now, will you get value from your investment?

Make progress, don't perfect mistakes

If you are going to learn what you need to do to make regular progress, it is critical to do a regular *written* review of your training, nutrition, rehabilitation, and other parts of your fitness program.

Most people don't do this. That is one reason that you see many people who are diligent about doing their training never making much or any progress once they get past the first few months.

If you get into the habit of doing monthly reviews you can learn what is working for you and not working. When you know what is not working you can begin crafting strategies to make needed changes in what you are doing.

I'm not exaggerating when I say that in the 60+ years I have been going to gyms, a sizable majority of people doing workouts hit a plateau in the first year or so *and never get any better.* I have seen people stuck year after year never getting any stronger, still trying to lose that "last 10 pounds" or wondering why they can't do certain movements.

In virtually every case these people have never attempted to evaluate the reasons for their continuing plateaus. They are going through the motions of working out but can't seem to get beyond a certain point.

Not correcting mistakes is a little like repeating 4th grade over and over. If you don't know what you are doing wrong, you can't make corrections and are bound to repeat the error indefinitely!

That is why I *strongly recommend* doing a monthly review of your progress. You should do this every month. This review is extremely important in helping you learn what you need to know to reach your fitness goals.

You are investing many hours in training and focusing on your nutrition. If you are going to get the maximum payoff from your effort, it behooves you to understand what is working and what is not working the way you would like. In other words, if you put in the time and effort, you should get the benefit.

Review format

It is important to do your review *written on paper.* If the review is not on paper, it is like writing messages on beach sand. As soon as a wave breaks over them, they vanish.

For a review to be on any value to you it must be enduring. Written records are the only format where you can be assured that your evaluations will be preserved.

Relying on memory is a very bad idea. Few people can recall the details of their last workout let alone detailed assessments of their month to month progress over a long time period.

The assessment itself is straightforward. It is divided into reviews of your training practices and your nutrition practices. If you are doing rehabilitation, this should be included as well.

The format I have used for decades is as follows:

Workouts

What is working well?   (based on goals and vision)

Why does this appear to be working?

What milestones did I reach this month?

What is NOT working?

Why? (if you know)

Outside help needed? (who, etc.)

Nutrition

Is this going according to plan?

Problems or issues

What is NOT working

Outside help needed?

Action Plan to Correct Deficiencies

Workouts

Nutrition

This is not like trying to learn thermodynamics. It is a simple format to help you get needed feedback from your hard work so that you can get the results you want.

I recommend that you do this evaluation on the last day of each month so that you can make needed changes to your program beginning on the first day of the new month.

Remember: The Overwhelming Power of Persistence

If there is one trait of successful people in any pursuit it is persistence. Nothing of substance or value can be accomplished without persistence. This quote from Calvin Coolidge is worth repeating again:

> ...Nothing in the world can take the place of Persistence. Talent will not; nothing is more common than unsuccessful men with talent. Genius will not; unrewarded genius is almost a proverb. Education will not; the world is full of educated derelicts. Persistence and determination alone are omnipotent....

There is no area of endeavor where this applies more strongly than physical fitness. No one has ever accomplished anything in the physical realm simply by "showing up" and doing a little

The power of Concentrating on What you are doing

In your training, every workout is about mastering the skill of strength. You don't make progress toward proficiency by simply "showing up" and then "flopping and thrashing" through a workout.

To that end, in the course that follows you should think of each training session as an opportunity to get better at something, work on your skills, and build up your capabilities.

Mastering anything requires concentrating on what you are doing. When you do a workout, you should be thinking and concentrating on what you are doing, not on the music in your headset or the tv monitors positioned above the treadmills.

You wouldn't try to learn something very complicated such as playing the piano, flying an airplane, or driving a race car while you were distracted by music playing in ear phones or having your attention diverted. Learning what you need to do requires *all* your concentration.

The same is true in physical fitness training. You need to have all your attention focused on what you are doing. If your mind is distracted by outside stimuli, you won't be able to learn what you are supposed to be doing.

I you want to master something, even the most elementary activity, eliminating distraction is essential.

Get rid of the ear buds, cell phones, and tv monitors during your training. Focus on how every movement feels, how every rep feels. To make serious progress, you must fully engage your mind to support the development of your physical capabilities.

Doing each weight lifting movement requires developing and refining different lifting skills. Each time you train, you should consciously focus on how to do the movements perfectly. This is the path from unconscious incompetence to conscious competence.

Developing the habit of being focused on what you are doing on every exercise and every movement will be critical in developing your skills of strength and your ability to master difficult movements.

Don't fall into the trap of distracting yourself during workouts. Distracted people are those who are usually "going nowhere but doing it to music".

Month

3

"I am not the product of my circumstances, I am the product of my decisions"

- Steven Covey

"Too many of us are not living our dreams because we are living our fears"

-Les Brown

Month 3

Weight training: Power Foundation

Ready for Month 3

You are now two months into your reconditioning program. You have probably begun to feel the benefits of being in good shape all the time. You feel stronger; your body feels alive, you walk differently, you have more zest and energy than when you started. A lot of subtle but significant things.

This is what the everyday life of a fit individual "feels" like.

By now you may not even think about whether you can do tasks of everyday life such as carry groceries, climb stairs, or move furniture, and lift heavy stuff…for fun.

Your endurance, athleticism and durability have improved dramatically. Now it is time to focus on building strength and lean muscle mass.

By now you have completed eight weeks of training to build up your muscular endurance and resilience. With the first two months of preparation, you can now go into the strength building phase of the program.

What's New this Month?

In the first two months of the program, you learned (or became re-acquainted) with several weight training exercises, and basic cardiovascular conditioning. With this foundation, you are ready to take on some more difficult training.

This month the core of your weight training will be on using the "Big 3" power exercises to develop what is called "whole body strength". Performing the bench press, squat and deadlift will activate almost every muscle in your body on each repetition.

You are now in significantly better condition that you were at the start. This means you can train harder. At the end of each session you should feel ready to do more. The big difference will be that you will be able to use weights that may have been completely out of reach when you started.

A significant change from the first two months is that you will be doing *four training sessions a week* instead of three. You will train on two days back to back with a day of rest in between. You will do slightly fewer exercises but done with more intensity.

The actual days you choose to do this are up to you, but I'll write about them as if you trained Monday-Tuesday and Thursday-Friday.

The exercises will be split between primarily upper body work on Monday and Thursday, and lower body work on Tuesday and Friday.

You will also be introduced (or re-introduced) to interval aerobic training. It involves doing periods of intense exertion followed by "recovery" periods of a specific duration.

For example, a 40-second sprint could be followed by a 20 second recovery period. This pattern would be repeated a planned number of times.

The effect of this pattern is to rapidly build aerobic capacity, overall fitness, and endurance. It can also be an effective for fat loss if the person is in halfway decent condition.

Interval training was introduced in the 1936 Olympic Games as a training program for sprinters. Following World War II, almost every track athlete in the world began using some form of interval training depending on the distance they ran.

Interval training remains the backbone of virtually all competitive running workout programs. Runners (and swimmers, and cyclists, etc.) at all levels from world class athletes to week end competitors use interval training as a mainstay in their workouts.

Back in my youth when I was a sprinter in track, I used a variety of interval training programs. As I aged, and moved into longer distances, I continued to use interval training to promote speed and endurance.

Today at age 78 I still use interval training in my own aerobic workouts.

As you can see, interval training can be adapted to almost anyone's training needs. That is why I'll introduce it to you at this point in your reconditioning.

Sets, reps, and weights

Up to now you have been doing exercises doing anywhere from 6-10 repetitions. This month you will be doing some of the exercises for only 5 repetitions per set.

On the five rep sets you will be using heavier weights than on higher rep sets.

How do you decide what weight to use?

Experiment to see what weight you can use where the final rep of the set is modestly difficult.

On the exercises that you do for five reps, you will increase the weight on each set. The general rule is the first set will be the lightest and the third set will be the heaviest.

The idea is that you start with a weight you can do 5 reps with relatively easily and progress to the last set where you must put out about 85% effort to get the last rep completed.

Over the month of training you gradually increase the weight you are using on all the sets. At the end of the month your starting set may be with a heavier weight than you could have used on your final set at the beginning.

The idea is to gradually increase the weight as your body gets stronger. Your body will adapt to small regular increases. These small increases add up to big increases over time.

One thing to always remember. Progress will only come if you work with weights that are not too close to your limit.

This is Dan John's "easy strength" principle. If you train below your limit, you will get progressively stronger. You will exceed your old maximum lifts by regularly increasing your sub-maximal training poundage's.

Even though you will focus on building "strength", you won't be doing anything like a maximum lift. You should never exceed what you believe to be an 85% exertion level.

There are multiple reasons for this. First, your muscles will grow stronger if you keep your exertion at 85% than if you try to go "all out". Your "85% effort" will increase steadily, whereas if you try to go at 100% you will quickly stop improving.

This is the dreaded "plateau" where many lifters spend most of their training lives.

This is because your body is still reestablishing the neuro muscular connections that will allow you to put out full power on any lift. You are also in the process of rebuilding your muscle density, and the resilience of your connective tissues.

Begin with weights that require you to put out about 85% effort on the final rep of each set. You can increase the weight you are using when all reps feel well within your capability.

Exercise Groupings

Day #1- (Monday and Thursday)

   Warm ups: Arm circles and scorpion

1. Bench press (3 sets 5 reps)
2. Push Press (3 x 5)
3. Barbell curl (3 x 5)

4. Deadlift (3 x 5)
5. One arm rowing (3 x 5)
6. Upright rowing (3 x 5)
7. Skull crusher (3 x 5)

Aerobic training follows weight training.

Day #2 (Tuesday and Friday)

Warm ups: unweighted squat and good morning exercise

1. Goblet squat (3 x 5)
2. Barbell squat (3 x 5)
3. Lunge with dumbbells (3 x 5)
4. One hand kettlebell swing (3 x 10)
5. Barbell rowing (3 x 5)
6. One hand farmers walk (2 x 50-foot walk)
7. Pushups (3 x 5-10)

Aerobic training follows the weight workout.

Weight Training – Day #1

1. **Bench Press**

Bench Press: You have been practicing this movement for several weeks now, so I'll limit the amount of instruction included here.

This month you will do the bench press for **3 sets of 5 reps.**

The main difference between how you may have been bench pressing up to now and how you should press in **do *a pause while holding the bar on the chest for the first two reps of the five-rep set.***

Take the bar off the rack, take a deep breath, and hold it. Then lower the bar to the bottom of your chest.

After pausing the bar at the bottom of the bench press, exert full power to drive the bar back up to the starting position. Exhale when the bar is ¾ of the way back to the starting position.

Do the pause only on the first two reps of a five-rep set.

2. Push Press

This movement is like a one arm dumbbell press, only you "cheat" by bending your knees and then driving the weight upward by quickly straightening them.

Because of the leg drive, you can use a heavier dumbbell than you could if you were doing a strict press. At first select a weight that is about 5 pounds heavier than one you would use for a strict standing press.

You can use either a dumbbell or a kettlebell in this lift.

Begin by bringing the weight to your shoulder. Hold it in place and take a deep breath. Hold the breath while you flex your knees and drive the weight to arm's length. When your arm is fully extended, drop the weight back to your shoulder. Don't release your breath until the weight has come back to the starting position at your shoulder.

In this exercise you are training your body to absorb the shock of the weight dropping down (under control) from arm's length. You will want to hold your breath to help absorb the shock of the weight dropping down to the starting position.

Part of the training effect of this lift is to begin conditioning your body to absorb a variety of shocks. It will also train you to control heavy objects above shoulder level.

Overall, this is one of the movements that will enhance your balance, coordination, and overall body control.

You should begin with a weight that you can control easily for five repetitions with each hand. Gradually work up to lifting a weight that gives you a little challenge on the final rep.

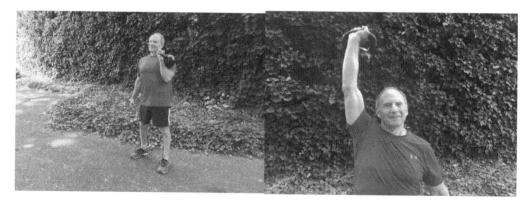

Starting position for push press and arm fully extended

Do 3 sets of 5 reps.

3. Barbell Curl

Your biceps get involved any time you lift, grasp, or pull something. Besides being a prime "t-shirt" muscle, the biceps muscles are super important to your overall strength.

There are many variations of this movement. In this month's program you will use the barbell version of the curl.

Begin with the barbell at arms length in front of you. Your grip should be with palms facing forward. Take a deep breath and hold it. Tighten your abdominal muscles, legs and glutes. Keep them tight while you do this exercise.

Using strict form and focusing on the muscles in your arms, slowly bring the barbell up to your neck.

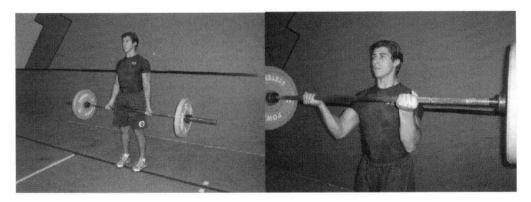

Barbell Curl: Start position and halfway to top position

When you have brought the weight to your neck, gradually release your breath, and lower the weight slowly to the starting position.

It is important to use strict form on this exercise. Many people "cheat" by beginning the lift with partially bent arms or generating momentum with their hips to drive the barbell upward.

Doing the exercise with strict form will give you arm strength through the full range of motion

Do **3 sets of 5 repetitions in the curl.**

4. Deadlift

This is one of the "big 3" power exercises that will be at the core of this program and your long-term conditioning.

Maximizing your potential will require that you master proper technique for this lift.

Like the squat and bench press, most of the deadlifts you see done in a gym will be performed with atrocious form. Vanishingly few trainers have any idea how to do this lift. Most people doing workouts mimic what they think they have seen.

Like the other power lifts, many of the most important parts of deadlift technique occur inside the body, out of sight of most observers.

You should carefully study the instructions here to start doing your deadlifts correctly on the first day you train with them.

The first step for good technique for the lift begins with proper set up. The bar should be resting on the floor in front of you. Walk up to it until your shins are touching the bar. Your feet should be 8-12 inches apart.

Take a deep breath and hold it. Keep your back flat as you lower your hips down so that you can grasp the bar at the same width as your shoulders. Your abdominal muscles should be tight as you go down to grip the bar.

You will grip the bar with one hand palm facing forward, and the other hand palm facing you.

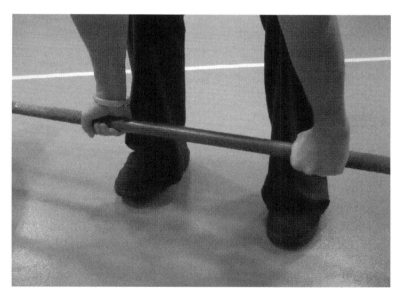

Deadlift Grip

Your entire body should be tight as you lower your hips to the starting position. Never make the mistake of being relaxed when you do your set up. When you are ready to pull, your body should be fully flexed.

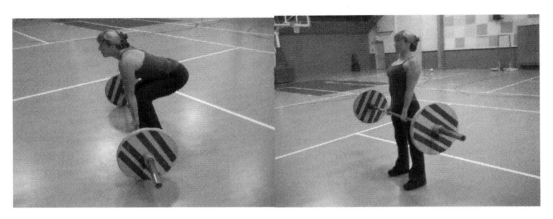

Deadlift – Starting position and finishing position

Roll your shoulders back, and have your head erect when are in the starting position.

When you are in the starting position, pull upward with about 50 pounds of pressure before you move the bar off the floor. This technique is critical if you are going to be able to maximize your strength. When the weights get heavy, applying upward force before moving the bar will be essential if you are going to make limit lifts.

When you begin the pull off the floor, you should keep your hips down and your back flat. Your back should be flat throughout the entire lift. NEVER allow your shoulders to round over. Keep your head erect and your back flat.

You will know you are pulling properly if you feel the lift in your abdominal muscles and hips. If you feel it in your lower back, your butt is raised up too high.

Keep the bar tight against your body as you pull. Keep your shoulders back.

When you are standing erect, square your shoulders, push your chest out and release your breath.

Lower the bar back to the floor *under complete control.* The bar should land on the floor with barely a sound. You should take a deep breath on the way down so that you are completely tight when the weight is again on the floor. You are now ready for your next rep.

A few comments on the current practice of slamming the bar down on the floor after completing a lift. First, dropping the bar is something that is only OK in competitive Olympic style competitive lifting. People in Cross-Fit gyms sometimes drop the bar when they are using rubber bumper plates. IMHO dropping the bar is never OK in any other circumstance. It should be lowered and *placed* back on the floor.

My observation over the past few years is that dropping the bar is usually done by minimally competent lifters who have mastered dropping weights to draw attention to themselves. Unless you are doing Olympic style lifting, dropping weights is a good way to look like a fool.

You should do 3 sets of deadlifts with 5 reps per set.

5. One Arm Rowing

Begin by placing your left knee on a bench. Bend over and place your left hand on the bench. Your right foot should be on the floor.

Take a dumbbell at arms' length in your right hand. Take a deep breath and pull the dumbbell up to your waist using your back muscles (lats) to do the lifting. When the dumbbell is at your waist, release your breath and slowly lower the weight back to the starting position.

Pull the dumbbell up to your waist in a smooth motion. Make your lat muscles do all the work. Don't jerk the weight or use your body to generate momentum.

Use a relatively heavy weight. You will do 3 sets of 5 reps with this exercise.

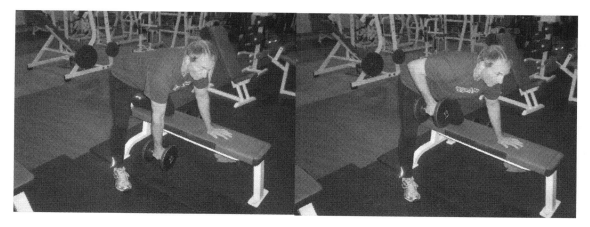

One hand dumbbell row: starting and top position

6. Upright Rowing

Grasp a barbell with a grip slightly narrower than shoulder width. Stand erect and let the barbell hang at arm's length in front of you.

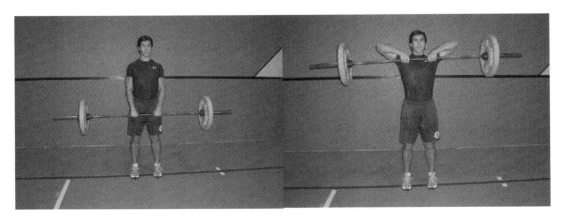

Upright rowing: starting position and top position

Take a deep breath and hold it. Smoothly pull the barbell up to a point where it is at the level of your collar bones. Slowly release your breath and gradually lower the bar to the starting position at arm's length in front of you.

Keep the movement smooth and under control. Do not jerk or use your body to generate momentum to the bar.

Do for 3 sets of 5 receptions.

7. Skull Crusher

This is a charming name for an exercise that will build real power in your triceps.

Begin lying prone on an exercise bench. Take a barbell (long or short) in both hands with your hands roughly 12 inches apart. When you set up on the bench, the barbell should be lying on your chest, so you can steady yourself on the bench.

Keep your feet flat on the floor, have a slight arch in your back, and push your shoulders into the bench.

When you are completely steady on the bench, push the bar to arm's length over your chest. Take a deep breath and hold it.

Keeping your elbows pointing straight up at the ceiling, lower the bar toward your forehead. The work in this lift should be done entirely by your triceps.

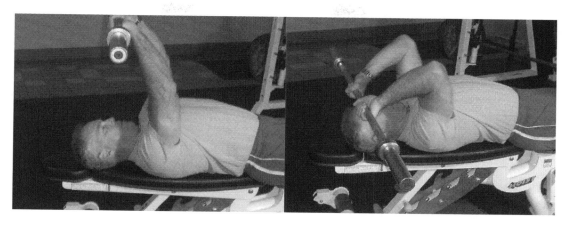

Skull crusher: starting and finishing positions

When your hands touch your forehead, push the bar back to the starting position.

It is essential that your elbows point upward throughout this exercise. You are isolating the triceps muscles and want them to do all the work in this movement.

If you drop your elbows and do a close grip bench press, you won't get the intended benefit from the movement.

Do 3 sets of 5 reps.

Day #2 – Weight Training (Tuesday and Friday)

Warm Up Movements

The highlight of the second day's weight training will be doing squats. To get maximum benefit from this exercise, it is important to be warmed up and ready to lift.

The overhead squat and good morning stretch will be warm up movements done with either an empty bar or a lightweight stick. The intent is to do the full range of motion and get rid of any stiffness you may have from the previous days training.

Overhead squat

This movement stretches your entire body, with emphasis on the hips, back and legs. It mimics an Olympic style snatch but is done without weight. Use a broomstick, pvc pipe or a wooden dowel rather than a barbell.

Stand upright holding the wooden dowel over your head. Extend your hands out in either direction so that you have a grip on the dowel that is wider than your shoulders by a foot or more on each side.

Holding the dowel over your head, descend into a deep squat. Keep the dowel directly over your head, or slightly behind your head.

When you have gone into a full squat, return to a standing position while holding the stick overhead. Do ten repetitions.

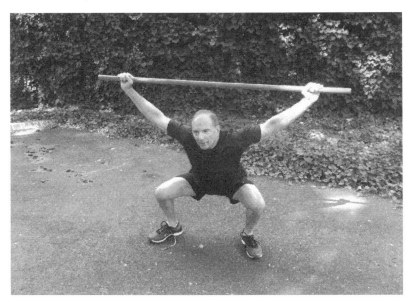

Overhead squat

Some people may find that it is difficult to get into deep squat position with your arms extended overhead. If this is the case, work over time to *gradually* increase the depth of your squat. This movement is very important in helping you develop a flexible body capable of a full range of motion.

Good Morning stretch

The first is a stretch movement with an empty barbell on your back. It is called the "good morning" exercise. In advanced training programs it is done with heavy weights to build massive strength in your posterior power chain.

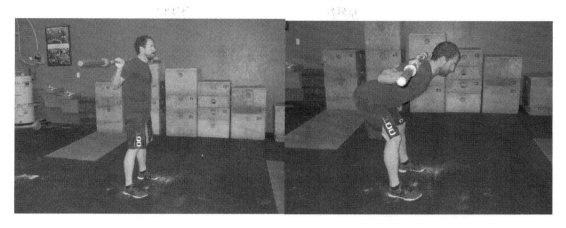

Good Morning Stretch

In the warm up version, place a barbell across your shoulders as if you were going to squat. Then bend forward at the waist, keeping your legs and back straight. Go to a point where you can feel a light stretch in your lower back and hamstrings. Hold in the low position for a count of two then return to the upright position.

Do not allow your back to round over at any point. Keep tight abdominals when bending forward. You should never force the stretch. The intent is to get your body ready to lift, not move a heavy weight.

Day #2- Weight Training

1. **Goblet Squat**

The goblet squat will train your body through a full range of the squatting motion. This lift will not only build leg strength, it will do wonders for your core strength, your back, shoulders and the rest of your body. It is one of those lifts that is great for your overall strength and athleticism.

This is easiest to do with a kettlebell but can also be done with a dumbbell.

Begin standing erect holding a single kettlebell by the handles just below your chin. Stand erect with your feet shoulder width apart. If you use a dumbbell, grab the weight by one end and hold it in front of your chin.

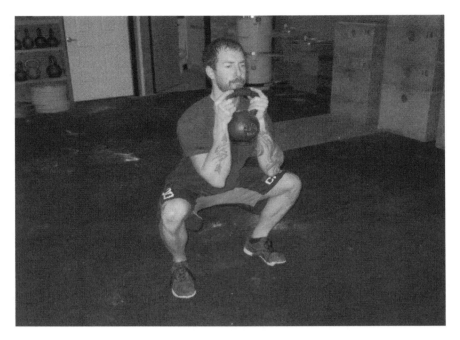

Goblet squat – bottom position

At the start, your elbows will be pointed down, and your forearms against your chest.

Take a deep breath and hold it. Begin squatting down by pushing your butt back as if you were going to sit in a chair.

As you slowly descend you should keep your shins as vertical as possible. Keep your chest up and your back flat. Do not ever allow your knees to bend outward past your toes.

Descend into the deepest squat you can manage. It may take some time, but you goal is to restore your full range of motion. Working on "going deep" with the goblet squat will do wonders to restore the strength and flexibility to your hips and legs.

2. Barbell Squat

The squat is one of the greatest exercises ever devised for building strength, power and athleticism. However, it is one of the least popular lifts anywhere.

Why?

Because it is *hard.*

In this program, I'll introduce you to the squat with the belief that you will work on it with zeal and perseverance. If you do, I promise you will find that your overall body strength will grow exponentially.

The squat requires a lot of attention to proper technique. As this may be your first exposure to the squat, I'll give you the basic pointers on good technique with the caveat that to really excel at this lift, you will have to master the technique. You can find detailed guidance on perfect technique in my books *Mastering the Squat* and in *Powerlifting Over 50*.

The most important first step in doing a good squat is the get the bar placed properly on your back. In my many decades going to gyms, I can assure you that close to 98% of people attempting to do the squat screw this up.

The bar needs to be placed across your upper back as shown in the photo below.

Almost everyone you see in a gym will put the bar up on their neck. This puts a heavy weight directly on the thinnest and most vulnerable part of your upper body. The bar rests on your neck vertebra. To compensate for this, many people will use a pad or wrap a towel around the bar.

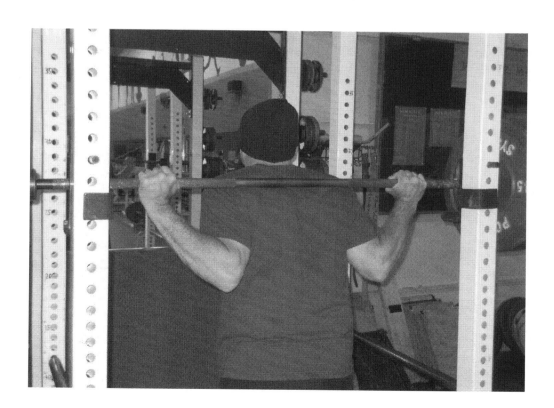

The high bar position is an all-around bad idea. Placing the bar this high is both dangerous and self-limiting. The risk of injury is high, and the weights you can use are artificially low.

The bar placement in the picture above shows the weight secure across the shoulders. This is the thickest and strongest part of your upper body. That means when you push up from the bottom position of a squat you are putting pressure on a wide muscular area rather than a narrow vulnerable area.

For your own safety, I strongly recommend that you always squat in a power cage like the one shown in the picture. That way if you are unable to complete the lift, you can put the weight on the support bars shown at the bottom of the picture.

When you position the rack height I *always* recommend that you set the rack height so that you will have to bend your knees to get under the bar. Setting the rack height so that you must lift upward to remove the bar from the rack means that it will be both easy to lift off and easy to return to the rack after you lift.

If you struggle on tip toes to get the bar back on the rack supports, you are asking for a big accident.

Once you have loaded the bar and are ready to take it off the rack, position it on your back as shown above. Then stand up and pause for a second or two to insure the weight is balanced on your back and you have it under full control. If it is not stable, put it back in the rack immediately.

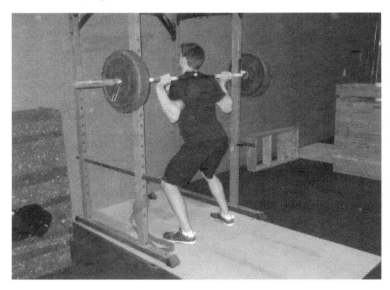

Proper position for taking the bar off the rack

In the photographs I have the model with their back to the camera to show proper bar position, rack height, and foot spacing. *When you do the lift, <u>face in the opposite</u>*

direction. You should always be stepping backward to do the squat, and forward to place the bar back on the rack.

When the weight is stable on your back, *take one step back from the rack*, and then bring your other foot back so that you are standing erect with your feet slightly wider than shoulder width.

Your head should be erect, your gaze straight ahead. Tighten your entire body!!!! Have a very tight grip on the bar.

Take a deep breath and hold it. Begin your descent by pushing your butt back as if you were sitting in a chair. Keep your shins as straight up and down as possible.

As you go lower into the squat position, push your knees outward so that your shins remain vertical.

Keep your back flat throughout the lift. Never roll your shoulders over

Keep your chest up as you go into the deeper position. That way your hips will go lower, and you will avoid the serious mistake of sticking your butt up in the air.

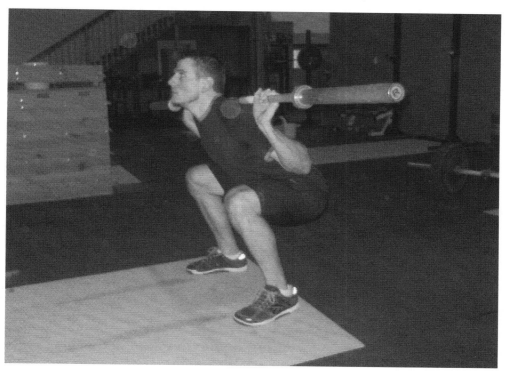

Proper body position in the deep part of a squat.

You will notice the knees are aligned with the toes. If the knees get forward of the toes, it puts tremendous strain on the knees and patella tendon. It is also a very unstable position and thus risky.

In the deepest part of the squat you will still be holding your breath. Your full lungs will give you something to push against as you begin to drive upward out of the bottom of the lift.

Once you get to the deepest part of the squat, immediately begin to drive upward.

You should come out of the bottom of the squat using the same body alignment that you had when you descended. Your chest should be up and lead the rest of your body out of the bottom.

A common mistake is making the first move upward by elevating your hips. This gives you a nose down and tail up configuration which places a lot of strain on your back. It can also lead to you losing control of the weight.

Keep your back flat and your abdominal muscles tight during your return to the starting position.

When you are about ¾ of the way back to the standing start position you can release your breath.

You should complete the squat by standing completely erect with no bend in your knees and chest up. At this point you can take in a deep breath and do another repetition.

Do 3 sets of 5 repetitions

3. Lunge with dumbbells or kettlebells

After you complete your squats, the lunge movement should be done at a lesser intensity. Concentrate on doing a full range of motion and don't be too concerned about the amount of weight you use.

Lunges help build strength and flexibility in your legs, hips and back. It also helps develop balance and coordination.

Take a dumbbell or kettlebell in each hand. Stand with your feet roughly 6 inches apart. Take a deep breath and hold it. Lift your right foot and move it *straight back* until your toe contacts the floor a few feet behind you. At the same time allow your left leg to bend into a partial kneeling position. Hold the weights in your hands at your sides.

Stand upright from this kneeling position by *straightening your front leg.* Bring your back foot up to the starting position. Release your breath. You should be standing in the same spot where you began the exercise.

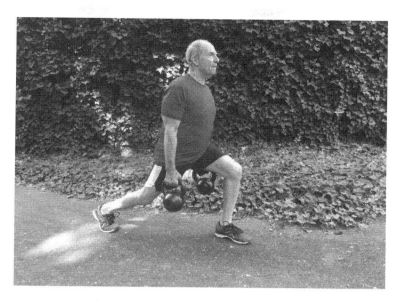

Lunge

Now extend the left foot behind you and do the movement. **2 sets of 5 reps with each leg**.

4. One hand Kettlebell swing

You have been doing the two-hand kettlebell/dumbbell swing already. Now you will begin doing the one hand swing.

Start with the weight on the ground in front of you. Take a breath and hold it. Bend your knees to get down so

that you can extend your arms and grasp the weight with your right hand. Keeping your back flat, head erect, and shoulders aligned over your knees, swing the weight back between your legs as if you were hiking a football.

Quickly straighten your legs and drive the hips forward until you stand erect. Pinch your glute muscles together as you reach the top of the swing. At the top of the swing, you should be standing upright and not leaning back with your arm parallel to the ground.

Release your breath as the weight approaches the top of the swing. Quickly inhale again as the weight begins to descend.

As the weight descends, bend your knees, and allow momentum to carry the weight back into the "hike" position. You should be holding your breath with tension in your abdominal muscles at the lowest point in the lift.

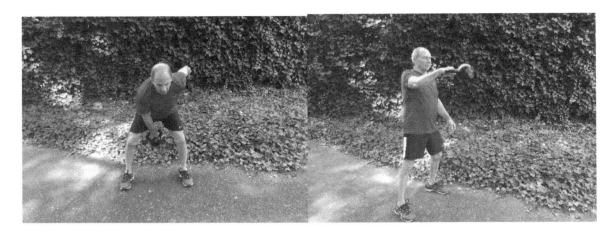

One hand swing – going to "hike" position   One hand swing – top position

Perform 2 sets of 8 repetitions with each hand. Begin with the right hand, and do 8 reps. Switch the weight to the left hand and do 8 reps. That is one set.

You will gradually increase the repetitions until you can comfortably do 12 reps with each hand. At that point, increase the weight and drop back to doing 8 repetitions.

Try to keep the time you spend recovering between sets to 60 seconds.   If that is too hard, use a lighter weight.

5. Barbell Rowing:

Start with the barbell on the floor in front of you. Stand so that your shins touch the bar, with your feet a bit wider than shoulder width.

Bend over and grasp the bar with the same width of grip you would use in the bench press. Keep your back flat and just above parallel to the floor. Keep your head slightly up to prevent any rounding in your upper back.

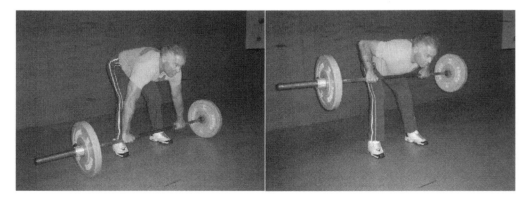

Barbell Rowing – Start position and top position

Take a deep breath and hold it. Pull the bar up to your waist.

When the bar is at your waist, pause for one second, release your breath and lower the bar under control back to the starting position.

This should be almost the exact opposite movement you just did in the bench press. You are using the antagonist muscles to the ones you used in the bench press. For example, you are using your biceps to pull the bar upward instead of the triceps to push the bar upward.

Do **3 sets of 5 repetitions.**

6.   One hand farmers walk

Walking with a weight on one hand may seem like an unusual exercise, but you will quickly see this movement can do wonders for your conditioning.

Select a dumbbell or kettlebell that you can carry for roughly 50 feet. The weight should be heavy enough so that you must work to do the exercise, but not so heavy that you have difficulty walking 50 feet.

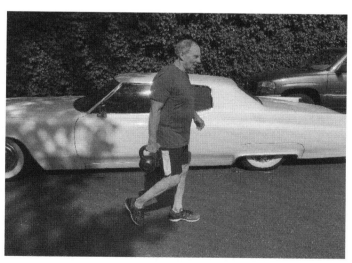

One hand farmers walk

With your arm at your side, take the weight in your right hand. Walk for roughly 50 feet and transfer the weight to your left hand. Walk back to your starting point.

This is a simple movement to describe, but it works a huge number of your muscles in the action of walking, and the fact that the weight you are holding is unbalanced between your left and right sides. This is a super training exercise for your core (abs, obliques, lower back, etc.).

Do three of these 50-foot walks with the weight in each hand.

7. Pushups

One of the best overall arm strength exercises is the pushup. It builds endurance and durability as well as solid muscle mass. People tend to overlook this exercise because it does not have the glamor of movements such as the bench press.

This is a "whole body" exercise that will enhance not only your strength, but your endurance and overall athleticism.

Begin by placing your palms on the floor slightly wider than shoulder width. Place your feet slightly wider than shoulder width and assume a position where you are supporting your body on the palms of your hands, and your toes.

If doing pushups from this position is too difficult, you can do them balanced on your knees instead of your toes.

Keep your body rigid throughout this exercise. Do not allow it to sag downward or put your butt in the air as you push up and down to the floor.

Lower your body until your chest is about 1" off the floor. As you lower yourself. your arms should be drawn into your sides. This will protect your shoulders from excess stress.

When you reach the bottom position, reverse the thrust and push your body back to the starting position.

You should keep your elbows in close to your sides for generating optimal thrust from your lats. This is essential for doing your best bench presses.

You can set your hand spacing wider after you are able to do 10 pushups with your hands spaced slightly wider than shoulder width.

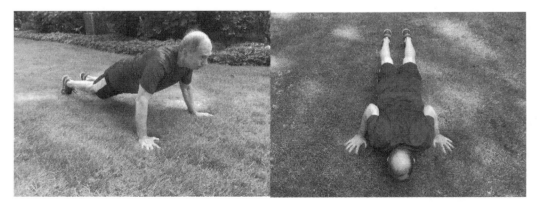

Starting position   Bottom Position

After you have built a solid foundation, you should do multiple sets of pushups with different hand spacings as part of your normal training.

In this program, begin by doing **3 sets of 5 pushups** and work up to the point where you can do **3 sets of 10**. Remember to stop the set when you are exerting more than 80% effort. By stopping short of your maximum, you will continue to progress.

Month 3: Aerobic Training - Timed Intervals

Intervals can either be for specific distances, or for specific times. In my opinion using specific times is the simplest way to begin.

For the trainee over age 50, there is some risk of doing intense exertion after being relatively inactive for years. For this reason, I emphasized developing aerobic conditioning with low intensity work in the first two months.

Unless you are already doing demanding aerobic training, you risk significant injury without going through a period of getting your body used to the rigors of interval training.

Intervals will give you a lot of return on your effort. But, your body must be ready to train this hard.

I'm recommending that your aerobic training consist of the following interval program in month 3:

Begin by warming up with a 50% effort pace for 2-3 minutes. This gets you ready to do the surges listed below.

1. Gradually accelerate over 3-5 seconds to an 80% effort pace – hold at 80% for 15 sec
2. Decelerate to 40-50% pace -hold for 60 seconds
3. Accelerate to 80% for 15 seconds
4. Decelerate to 40-50% for 60 seconds
5. Accelerate to 80% for 15 seconds
6. Decelerate to 40-50% for 60 seconds

This is one complete "set" of intervals.

If this is the first time you have done interval training, I strongly suggest that you begin with three interval sets and keep the intensity modest. Your body needs time to adapt to the intensity. If you feel three sets is not a challenge, you can add more interval sets if you feel (relatively) strong at the end of each set.

You see the interval pattern of high intensity (80% effort) lasts for 15 seconds and the recovery period at (40-50%) effort lasts for 60 seconds.

Don't exhaust yourself. You will make progress if you are working regularly within your capacity. Remember, you make progress with sub-maximal challenges.

Each person will progress at a different rate, so don't compare yourself to someone else. If you are making progress, that is what is important.

As you get in better condition, you can make your training more demanding by:

1. Adding more intervals (periods of high intensity effort and recovery)
2. Lengthening the period of high intensity (go from 15 sec to 20 sec, etc.)
3. Shorten the recovery period (go from 60 sec to 45 sec, etc)
4. Change the exertion period and keep the recovery the same (15-20-30 sec exertion and 60 sec recovery, etc.)

As you can see, interval training can be modified almost any way you choose.

Begin doing 3 interval sets and see work up to 5 sets by the end of the month.

Day #2- Aerobics (option)

At the end of the second day of back to back workouts, you may feel tired. For that reason, I'll suggest that *if you are feeling tired* you do a low intensity aerobic training session after the Day #2 weight training. Think of this as a "recovery" session.

Ten to fifteen minutes of jogging at a relaxed pace will help build your cardiovascular system, and not burn too much of your energy reserve.

If you feel you want to do more cardio, feel free to do so. However, remember you only have so much energy. The key to making progress is exercising AND recovering.

This is a challenging exercise program. When you finish this month's training you will be in dramatically better condition that when you began the program.

Your whole body will feel different, and your clothes may be loose in the waist and tight in the chest.

You have a taste of what it *feels* like to be strong and fit. You will be reconnecting with your physicality.

Nutrition: Month 3

Moving from "diet" to "lifestyle"

Your nutritional lifestyle is a key part of your vision of the fit person you are.

A nutritional "lifestyle" is something you have deliberately chosen. You are making conscious choices about what you are going to eat, how much and when.

What this means is that you are establishing a deep-rooted *practice of habitually* eating foods that make you fit and healthy. It comes naturally as breathing.

On the other hand, being "on a diet" is like holding your breath. You can do it for a while, but eventually you must take a breath. Diets are also a set of rules that most people see as being imposed from an outside authority.

"Diets" are temporary. Habitual eating patterns day in and day out are your "lifestyle".

As noted last month, diets, especially for fat loss, are something that people feel (consciously or unconsciously) is something they are *forced* to do. As soon as they don't *have to* comply with the diet, they go off of it…often in spectacular fashion.

Over the past two months you have been working on being very conscious of what you eat, why and how much. Presumably this has helped you be *in control* of what you eat and drink.

You shop for quality food, have it in your home, and don't eat crap.

When you make the best choices without thinking about it, then you have built good nutrition into your *lifestyle*.

At this point in your reconditioning you are defining your nutritional life style or how you intend to eat *for the rest of your life.*

A Dozen "Best Practices" to sustain a healthy nutritional lifestyle

First, establish an eating program that you will stay on, not one that is so difficult you won't have a chance of keeping on it for more than a couple of weeks.

I suggest that you experiment with different established eating programs such as the Paleo Diet, Mediterranean Diet, or Intermittent Fasting. You should see what works best for you and is a program you could stay with indefinitely.

Second, you should be aware that because you are over 50, your metabolism will have slowed so that you need less food than you did when you were 30. This is normal but is a factor that many people desperately want to ignore.

Like it or not, older people need less food than they did when they were younger.

Third, being hungry does not mean you should eat. Your appetite has little to do with what you need. It is a combination of genetics that kept our ancient ancestors hunting for food in the wilds, and mild addictions to sugar and salt.

If you feel hungry, ignore the pangs and stick with your plan. Your health and your appearance will reflect that.

Fourth, keep high quality nutritious food in your home. If you have "good stuff" available to eat, you won't have to deal with the temptation to eat junk.

Fifth, remember you can eat unlimited quantities of fresh vegetables and fruits. This does not include faux vegetables such as "corn" chips, deep fried chickpeas, or the myriad of other bagged delights.

Sixth, remember that alcoholic drinks are loaded with calories. You can subvert your nutrition plans with regular drinking. Despite what some of your friends might tell you, beer is not a vegetable, nor are grain-based liquors.

Seven, keep track of what you eat. That means write down what you ate, how much, and when. You can keep this data in a notebook, or on some device that will allow you to track everything that goes in your mouth.

Be aware that most people drastically underestimate how much they eat. Most studies show that even people who carefully record everything they eat, under estimate the quantity by half. In other words, before you write down that you ate "6 ounces" of something, actually weigh it out and see how accurate your estimate is. It is in your best interest to learn how to accurately estimate your food consumption.

Eight, there is a lot of really bad food out there that is packaged as "health food". The biggest offenders are baked goods you find in a coffee shop (eg. "breakfast" muffins, "whole grain breakfast bars", etc.) They are mostly sugar fats with a little artificial flavoring thrown in. They are genuinely terrible if you are trying to get (or keep) a lean muscular look. Many "Sports drinks" are basically a lot of sugar with caffeine added.

Remember, food vendors have no concern about what happens to you because of consuming their product, as long as you don't get sick or die suddenly. If you can barely get your pants zipped up because of eating too many "chippie dippies" or "jumbo fried sugar balls", don't blame the guys who sold you the stuff that made you fat.   You are their "target audience", and your mouth is a "business opportunity".

Nine, follow the "out of sight, out of mind" rule with junk food. Don't have it in your home. If junk food is right there where you can grab it any time, then it is a constant temptation for you. Remember, these foods were literally "engineered" to make you *crave* them…and eat more than you should.

I have already discussed the addictive properties of sugar. A lot of the "snack" foods you really don't want to have around are loaded with sugar. The food engineering process also uses salt and fat to make them more irresistible.

Ten, don't eat something because your bored or can't figure out what else to do. A lot of extra pounds go on people's butts because they eat mindlessly during the day or during the evening. Be fully aware of everything you are putting in your mouth. If it is not on your plan, don't eat it. You will wind up having it around your waist and will have to work it off before you put on your summer clothes.

Eleven, "food supplements" are not a substitute for eating properly. A lot of people seem to think if they take handfuls of pills (or powders), they can ignore eating properly. Dead wrong.

Far too many "supplements" are basically useless. Even the good ones are not intended to substitute for eating properly. I recommend a few "supplements" but strongly advise that you devote your time and money to getting your nutrition from food.

Twelve, build your nutrition around fresh food. That means vegetables that are sold raw. Meat, fish, eggs, dairy products and poultry are uncooked. Avoid things that come in a can, box or sealed bag.

Obviously, there are some exceptions to this (eg. Packaged butter, cheese, cured sausage, etc.). The key is to build your grocery shopping around minimally processed fresh food. Many frozen foods are excellent. You must take the time and expend the effort to learn what to buy.

There is no single "best diet"

Each person will respond to different eating programs slightly differently. You will be most successful if you spend the time finding out what works best for *you.*

What works best for me may not be something that will work for you.

The only way to find out what works best for you is to *experiment* with different programs.

It is really important that you continue to practice the good habits you began using in the first two months. You should always limit the amount of sugar you consume, minimize eating processed food, and stay far away from eating junk food.

This month, I'm suggesting that you begin experimenting with different eating "lifestyles". There are three that I strongly suggest you try for a minimum of two weeks to see how your body (and mind) respond.

I have used all of the programs listed here, so this is not an example of "do what I say, not what I do".

Each of them worked well for me, and I changed from one to another to find out how it impacted my body. Over time I have gradually evolved my own eating "lifestyle" that is a combination of a couple of these approaches.

It is my natural way of eating and living every day. I can eat properly without feeling like I'm making some type of sacrifice. In short, my instinct is to crave the things that are good for me.

The Paleo Diet

The simplest way to describe the Paleo diet is that you do not eat any grains or dairy. You eat fresh vegetables, fruit, meat, fish, nuts, eggs, and poultry. You do not eat processed food (can or box). In short, the essence of this program is to eat lots of veggies and fresh protein sources.

That is the *general* guidance. If you want to get into the fine details of the Paleo program, I suggest you check out the internet sources I have on my web site www.MidLifeHardBody.com.

If you want to experiment with the Paleo diet, try it for a few weeks. It may take that long for your body to adjust to the food and for you to feel comfortable eating that way.

The Mediterranean Diet

This program is based on eating fresh food and eliminating saturated fats (those solid at room temperature) and eating a diet high in monosaturated fats (eg. Olive oil). This diet is high in carbohydrates from fresh vegetables, fruit, seeds, nuts, and fish. This fiber rich diet includes minimal amounts of meat and dairy.

A two-week trial of this diet will give you a sense of how this program might work for you. Again, check the nutrition section of my web site for more information on this diet program.

Intermittent Fasting

Currently popular, this program involves limiting all food intake to one five to six-hour period during the day. You still eat "good stuff", but essentially do a fast for 18 hours between eating periods.

This approach is easy to implement. Simply select the time period when you will eat each day (example: 6-11 PM). Eat nothing (fast) all day until that time. During the fasting time it is OK to consume black coffee, water, or tea.

I use intermittent fasting as my own eating routine every day. After the first week, I never "get hungry" during the fasting period. I find that I have a good (but not ravenous) appetite when dinner time comes.

One thing that makes this approach more appropriate for older people than younger ones is that as we age our metabolism slows down about 1% per year past age 30. Thus, as more senior people we actually need less food to support our bodies than we did years ago. Eating less is what we are supposed to do.

Resources

If you go to my web site www.MidLifeHardBody.com, I have a list of nutritional guides to different programs that are available on line.

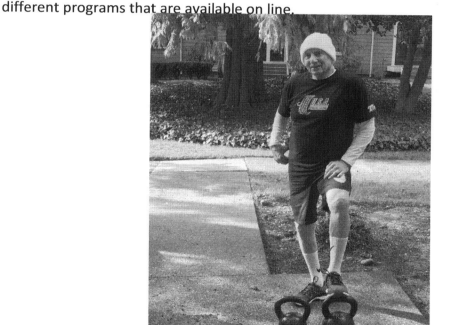

Mindset: Life Habits that Will REALLY help you

Nurture your vision of yourself as a fit person

Always remember, fitness is a journey not a destination. Embrace the idea that fitness is a *continuing lifestyle*, not just something like a vaccination that you do once and that is sufficient.

To sustain a fitness lifestyle, it is imperative that one develop *habits* that support and reinforce the good things you are trying to accomplish.

To get you started, here are some things you can do that will help you get the most return from your investment of time, money, and trouble. The list is not exhaustive, but it is a good place to begin.

These are:

Powerful life management habits

- Plan and execute the plan
- Manage your time -every day/week/month
- Always be persistent

Nourishing your mind and spirit

- Develop a "growth" mindset
- Seek out people who radiate positive energy
- Nurture relationships
- Workouts that are fun

Make your Plan then Execute

An unplanned life is the pathway to chaos. *If you have no plan, your plan is to fail!*

Your plan begins with your vision. The vision gets refined into goals. The more specific the goals are, the better the chance that they will be accomplished.

If you are new to an area, making a plan that is likely to work can be difficult. The programs in this book are your plan for getting back into good physical condition.

Your initial plan is to *do regular workouts as set forth in this book.*

Even the best plan is not worth much unless you *execute the plan.* "Doing" what is in the plan is where desired results come from.

Execution is where the hard work begins, and many people fall short.

The first requirement for successfully executing a plan is to develop and implement a schedule.

Time Management: Life on a Schedule

It is impossible to accomplish anything substantial without imposing the discipline (and power) of a schedule on your daily life.

People who have no schedule and allow outside events to dictate when they do things wind up at the end of each day having "gone like mad" and accomplished nothing. These people exhaust themselves doing an endless series of tasks that seem to require immediate attention. There are no clear priorities, only an endless parade of items on the "to do" list.

So...you should begin your quest to get back into super physical condition by setting up a *weekly* schedule. You are going to include all the things you *plan* to accomplish, and *when during the week you intend to do them.*

This means defining the time and place you intend to do each thing on your list.

One of the main reasons people fail at workout programs or doing anything that is not part of their existing routine, is that they have not scheduled a time and place where it will happen. When something has no place on the schedule, it means that it is not important enough to merit planning ahead.

So, begin by defining exactly when and where you will be doing your workouts.

Allocating your Effort

One of the recurring themes in books about how to be a more efficient and effective person is the power of managing the only resource they have that can never be made larger: time. Schedules basically define when certain things will occur during the day...every day.

Stephen Covey developed a powerful concept of time management that applies when thinking about health and fitness. (See *The 7 Habits of Highly Effective People*)

Inherent in time management is the idea that certain activities are *important,* and others are *not important.* *Important activities are those that produce results*. Examples of important activities would include developing a new skill, gainful employment, college courses, and of course physical fitness training.

Activities that are not important include a variety of things that produce no result. These would include watching television, most phone calls, social media exchanges, playing video games,

Each activity can be classified as either *urgent* or *not urgent*. Examples of an urgent event would be a phone ringing or a 911 type "crisis". Urgent activities require immediate attention. Activities that do not require immediate attention are considered not urgent.

The importance of an activity is not necessarily related to whether it is urgent or not urgent. In fact, most important activities, such as developing a job skill, getting fit, or enhancing your career, are activities things that a lot of require regular attention. However, in most cases these are not urgent, such as a ringing telephone or a crying baby.

Often the urgency of a task is not related to importance. In fact, most urgent activities are not important in that they produce no lasting result. Examples: most text messages, Tweets, most phone calls, etc.

In theory, important activities would be done instead of unimportant activities, but that is not how many people operate. Their days are consumed dealing with urgent (and not important) activities. They spend most of their day dealing with text messages, constant interruptions, and responding to whatever "crisis of the moment" appears.

If your objective is to produce lasting important results, you must schedule your life so that important activities get the most attention.

What you want to do is set yourself up to succeed, not set yourself up to fail.

Your workout time should not be encroached on by tasks that are not important. If something you do regularly is "not important" enough to be scheduled, quit doing it and put it out of your mind.

Now that you have *scheduled* your workouts, the next task is to do them and develop *useful documentation* of what you did each session.

Monitoring and Feedback: Staying on Course

To successfully execute your plan, it is an absolute requirement to keep track of what you are doing and how this activity is impacting your progress.

Everyone who trains seriously should keep *detailed* records of their workouts. This includes all your physical training, both weight training work, and aerobics.

A training plan is a specification of what you will do and when. In this phase of your training, you will use the workout plans in this book.

Without a detailed plan, you are basically doing random activity

To know if your plan is working, you need to accurately track what you are doing every workout over weeks and months.

It is imperative that everything be written down.

There are several reasons for this:

- It is impossible to remember detailed information on each workout (weights used, sets, reps, etc.) When following a training plan, it is essential that you know all of this to track how well you are doing on the program.
- In evaluating a training cycle, it is necessary to have data to determine what worked and what did not work.
- Detailed data is essential to track training volume and intensity.
- Successful training plans are based on hard data, not subjective evaluations or post-hoc guesses.

Begin with the date and time you do the workout.

Each workout should generate a big volume of data on what you do. For weight training this data will be the exercises, weights, sets and reps.   For aerobics, at minimum it will be what you did and for how long.

Every exercise and every set have an impact on your progress (or regression). This information should be easily available to you as you train over weeks and months.

This is much like getting in your car and saying you want to "go to Boston". If you don't monitor where you are, you have no clue whether you are going in the right direction, or in the opposite direction.

Important Records

The important information on your weight training workouts is:

- Exercise (eg. Standing press, squat, etc.)
  - Weight
  - Sets
  - Reps
  - Comments (hard, easy, awkward, problem with form, etc.)

For your aerobic training, the critical information is:

- Exercise (eg. running, cycling, etc.)
  - Duration (time or distance)
  - Pace
  - Comments (hard, easy, equipment issues, etc.)

Here is a hypothetical example of a weight training log:

Squat
        135 x 5 (135 lbs. for 5 reps) – easy warm up
        225 x 5 (225 lbs. for 5 reps) – focused on speed out of bottom
        275 x 5 (275 lbs. for 5 reps) – fifth rep becoming hard
        315 x 3 (315 lbs. for 3 reps) – focused on speed coming up
        275 x 3 (275 lbs. for 3 reps) – felt great finishing squats
                Comments: Could increase top weight by 5 lbs. next time

Here is a hypothetical example of an aerobics training log:

Treadmill
        Warm up pace – 5 min
        Alternate 30 second interval at 70% with recovery pace – 5 min
        Warm down pace – 5 min
Jogging
        2 miles @ 10-minute pace
Rowing Machine
        Warm up – 2 minutes
        Alternating 10 sec sprints with 50 sec recovery – 10 minutes
        Steady state row at 70% - 10 minutes
        Warm down – 1 minute

You may notice that all of the information included in the examples is about what you "do". This is the only training information that is of any real value.

A word of warning.

There are a growing number of very expensive gadgets on the market that measure many different fitness "parameters". These are things like "number of steps", "calories burned", "pulse rate", etc.

Estimates of "calories burned" or "heart rate range" are: 1) usually extremely inaccurate; or 2) of no real value unless you are in a hospital cardio rehab program.

However, they are the kind of measurements that software devices can easily track or estimate. *Because these data are easy to collect, that is what gets collected.*

Most of these "measurements" are basically useless to someone trying to get in shape. However, vendors develop slick looking devices to convince potential customers that the numbers these "apps" generate are important.

IMHO, this is a case where the cheap handwritten notebook is vastly better than the slick device that costs several hundred dollars.

A handwritten workout journal has major advantages over any of the commercial fitness trackers. These include:

- The amount of information available at a glance is huge.
- You can compare data on the same exercise from several different training sessions by simply turning pages
- You can compare work volume from workouts on different days at a glance
- You have notes about your performance on each exercise on a given day
- You can instantly assess whether you are improving according to your plan...or not.
- There is *no way* you can *easily* record and retrieve this information on a computer

I say this having been a "computer guy" for over 50 years. But, I have yet to find a fitness tracking "app" that is worth the time it takes to load on my i-Phone.

Persistence: The single most important factor for success

Everyone should ask themselves "what is the single most important thing a person must do to be successful?" The answer is *persistence.*

Remember the quotation earlier in this book. Nothing beats persistence; certainly not talent, education, or genius. These assets are squandered without persistence.

There is a natural human tendency to conserve energy. This was a useful survival mechanism for ancient humans who had to ready to escape predators or live on limited food supplies. In the modern world, our natural inclination leads to sloth, obesity, and poor health.

People are "out of shape" because they follow what comes naturally...conserving energy.

Getting "in shape" requires going against our natural inclinations.

The inclination to quit or backslide will be especially strong when you first start doing physical training again. Your body will tell you that you "need" to avoid running or lifting weights. Your mind must overcome this impulse.

Progress comes from regular practice; nothing else.

This applies whether you are studying physics or doing physical training. There is a direct relationship between the (physical and mental) effort you put in and the results you see.

If you are persistent, you will be rewarded.

Caring for the Mind and Spirit

The ancient Greeks always believed that a sound body and a sound mind were intimately intertwined. This is always good advice regardless of where you are in your life journey.

During my working life I was a PhD scientist (and manager) in a research and development company. When I retired from that gig, I did consulting for a venture capital firm, and some national security work.

After having a highly active and creative mental life for most of my years, I was not about to shut down the brain cells and blob out in front of the TV. Having a mental challenge was as important to me as having a physical challenge.

I got involved in working on line because it presented me with *part* of the mental challenge I need to stay happy and active from the neck up. If you mind dies, your body follow soon thereafter.

If your mind is active, you want to keep it that way.

It is really important that *you* constantly find things that keep you mentally challenged. Here are some thoughts on how to do this.

A Growth Mentality

You are never too old to try something new! Bank on this idea.

Many people believe that their personal potential is limited by the supposed "talent" they were given at birth. They believe that they are "smart" or "dumb", "a good athlete" or not, capable of learning math...or not. The list can go on and on.

One of the most common unexamined assumptions people make about themselves is "I'm not a very good at doing (fill in the blank)". Because a person *assumes* they can't do something, they never really question this assumption.

The power of these assumptions is that they effectively prevent you from trying something new or believing that you could accomplish something new and different *if you worked at it.*

You remember, this is called the *fixed mindset*. It is a killer of hopes and dreams.

The effect of limiting beliefs is that many people don't even try to do some things because they *assume* they will not succeed. As Henry Ford once said, "If you believe you can't do something, your right".

A critical point is that decades of research has shown that these beliefs about our own limitations are merely ideas we "believe" without testing them in the real world.

In real life it is impossible to predict is how far anyone can progress *if they work at being better.*

Clearly there are some limits, such as "learning" to play basketball well enough to play in the NBA or becoming a first chair violinist in a major symphony orchestra. But, a normal person can make huge advances in their life by believing they can do something, and *then working to make it happen!*

Your goal is to get back into shape after age 50. Begin by assuming that you have no idea how far you can go. You will make much more progress than if you begin by assuming you have some inherent limitation.

Embrace the *growth mindset.*

This is a very liberating idea. Through hard work you can *discover* what is possible for you.

Positive Energy around You

I'm not suggesting ignoring that bad things do occur. But, I have found that there is a big difference between being *realistic* about difficulties in life and *dwelling* on negative things.

You can be completely realistic about the difficulties and disasters of the world without carrying it around like a personal sack of woe. Being positive about your own life space will be refreshing and attractive to others. You will feel better too.

All of us have known people who go through life with an angry facial expression. They seem to be annoyed with everything.

We have also known people who always find something bad to say about whatever is going on. They are a "black cloud" on two feet.

These people *radiate* negative energy. This negative "force field" impacts everyone around them.

Don't hang around those types of people. In fact, stay as far away from them as you can.

Bring positive energy into everything you attempt, and you will be amazed at what happens.

If you want to see how a positive mood is contagious, try a simple trick.

When you walk down the street, or anywhere else you might encounter strangers, simply have a smile on your face. If you glance at someone with a smile, it is virtually impossible for them not to smile back.

Doing this you have conveyed positive energy in their direction and brightened their existence for a few moments. You are a like a beacon of light, rather than a walking "death star".

Here is another way to have a positive impact on people; ask them about what is going on with them. The late Dale Carnegie said that people will enjoy your company when you are "interested" in them as opposed to trying to be "interesting".

How many people do you know who go out their way to inform you about all the "fascinating" things they are doing rather than find out about what is going on with you? You probably don't feel any strong desire to be around them.

On the other hand, people who ask about what is going on with you, how you feel about things, and what you are thinking about are those you want to spend time with. You get the point.

If you radiate positive energy, people will be drawn to you.

Pursuing Excellence for the Right Reasons

One of the downsides of a high achieving life style is what psychologist Arthur Ciaramacoli called "performance addiction". This is a condition where certain individuals are constantly pursuing "perfection" in a given area to make up for some deficiencies they believe they have.

In *Curse of the Capable,* Dr. Ciaramacoli discusses high achievers who are driven by the belief that they can gain love and respect from various achievements. They feel inadequate and uncomfortable in their own skin.

The sad thing is that the harder these people work, they never seem to get "good enough" to feel good about themselves or get the rewards they really want.

If you have spent any time in a gym, you will probably have observed people who appear to be pursuing "the perfect body" or some variation on that theme. Their private logic seems to be that "If I'm perfect, then I will feel great and people will care about me".

The harder they try, the more elusive the reward. But, this just means they work harder. Life becomes a treadmill of constantly working harder for a satisfaction that never comes.

In this situation the persons motivation is *extrinsic.* They are driven by the belief that if they work hard enough they will be rewarded for their efforts from a source outside themselves.

The assumed opinions of other people have immense power over how they feel about themselves. They often compare themselves against arbitrary (and ever escalating) standards of perfection. The little voice in their head is constantly criticizing them for being inadequate in some way or another.

In short, being in their head is terrible because it is impossible to ever accomplish anything that is "good enough".

The opposite of this situation is when people take great care of themselves for the "right" reasons. These are people who accomplish great things *and enjoy doing it!*

Taking care of your body because it is something *you want to do* is *intrinsic motivation.* The reward comes from the feeling you get 24/7/365 from living in a body that feels good (and probably looks good).

People who honor themselves (and their family and friends) by *caring for themselves* find that they <u>*enjoy the process*</u> of training and being fit.

One way of illustrating this is an observation I have made about many competitive weight lifters. Rather power meets being the *reason* they work out; competitive events are an *excuse* to work out. The lifters would work out anyway, the meets just give them something to structure their training.

Taking care of yourself is a great idea. This is a benefit to you and everyone around you. But, using workouts as a hunt for "perfection" or to fill a hole in your life is a futile and potentially destructive pursuit.

There is nothing wrong with wanting to look great. There is probably something in our DNA that makes us want to be our best. The main thing is to give yourself "props" for having the guts to train hard even when it may be difficult and begin to feel the fun part of being physical.

Relationships

Building positive and nurturing relationships is essential to have a happy life. These are the bonds you build with people who are become close friends and intimate partners.

Building quality relationships, takes time and energy.

The first thing to ask about any relationship is whether it fills you with positive energy or whether it drains you. You should only keep or develop relationships that "fill you up". Avoid *any* relationships that drain you.

There are many choices in life that have consequences we may not fully appreciate at the time we make them. One of the biggest of these is who you associate with on a regular basis.

As you build relationships with others, think about the "Rule of 5". This means that you will take on the views and characteristics of the five people with whom you have the greatest amount of contact.

If you hang out with five negative people, you will be negative. If your 5 primary associates are poor people, you will probably become (or stay) poor.

Conversely, if you associate with positive energetic people, you will be positive and energetic.

If you associate with people who don't care about their health or fitness, or actively disparage working out, you will be pulled down by their negative energy.

On the other hand, if you work with a lot of people who are enthusiastic about getting fit or getting better at something, your performance will continually be elevated.

Essential point; your associates play a *huge* role in determining what you accomplish in life.

Building relationships that are deep and lasting can also take a lot of energy.

A key to building a good relationship is to be authentic. You can't build something solid and lasting if you can't be your *authentic* self. Many of us have been convinced that who we really are is not acceptable.

Being authentic should not be construed to mean focusing on all sorts of negative behavior or feelings. Many of us conceal our gentler and loving inclinations because it may not seem "cool", or we have built barriers between ourselves and other people.

Being authentic takes practice, and for many of us, a fair amount of courage.

Working Out for the Fun of it!

One of the most important things we can do in life is to have fun, to be joyful, to enjoy what we do.

Primitive man was programmed for survival. The modern desire to "have fun" is at odds with some of our more primitive human drives for survival. Our evolutionary heritage drove us to conserve energy in case we had to flee a predator, or search for food.

Over millennia, organized societies developed the security and abundance to permit expending energy on things that feel enjoyable, that are "fun", and none of those are a physical search for food or fleeing for our lives.

In fact, we now contend with an excess of food. And most of the predators we fled from are extinct or in zoos.

Still, humans are naturally designed for movement, if not for survival, per se, certainly for quality of life. Modern life circumstances dictate that we find ways to move in a culture and economy that requires little taxing physical activity.

When we were kids we spent our time "playing". Physicality was a big part of our play. We ran, we climbed, we explored. Play was doing a lot of things that didn't have rules. We did them because it felt good just to be doing them, because they were fun.

Fun is characterized by enjoying the process of "doing" whatever it is we are doing. We are in the moment, and feeling a range of emotions such as exhilaration, satisfaction, challenge, and joy.

While we may have a goal in mind, the feeling of fun is that what we are doing is inherently enjoyable. We would do the activity even without the goal.

If you think of physical training as "play", and working out as "fun", then the payoff for what you are doing is the workout itself, not finishing the workout. In other words, enjoying the *process*, not focusing on the goal or reward.

I have often thought that portraying workouts as a cross between Marine Boot Camp and sado-masochism was completely misguided. This creates the idea that if something is good for you, it is necessary to *force* yourself to do it.

Rubbish!

Make physical training part of your personal ecosystem of fun. Think it terms of "challenge", "satisfaction" and self-defined rules. You set the terms of what you do and enjoy the *process.*

Doing the workout is fun. The goals you have are there to guide what you do.

That is not to say that workouts should not be difficult, demanding and require hard work. The important thing is how you *experience* them.

For example, when I was doing heavy weight training, I always felt an inherent joy in "lifting heavy stuff". Before getting to the gym, I couldn't wait to start lifting. I still have this feeling of joyous anticipation for all the workouts I do.

Contrast this experience with "being on a diet".

Most people regard being on a diet as something to be endured. You constantly deny yourself things you want. Your mental focus is on what you *can't have.*

If you look at workouts as something you "should do", almost all your focus is on getting through them; eg. "can I stop now?"

When we were kids, it never occurred to us to stop playing until we *had* to. Now that we are adults, many of us have problems believing that we can *play* and have fun.

Physical training is something that can be a lot of fun. When you begin to think about workouts as "play time", you can begin to tap into the fun side of physical activity.

Live for today and tomorrow

All of us have a past. The past is done with and can never be changed.

A person's past can often be an anchor to living in the present and looking toward the future. You can change this by not letting your past corrupt how you think about your future.

The reality of our existence is that we only have the moment in which we are living...meaning *right this instant.* How we choose to live in this moment is up to us. We also have the future which has yet to be lived.

Your Next Steps

Congratulations! You have a great start on building a body that will give you a great quality of life for many decades. You have completed three months of physical training and are now well on the way to getting into great physical condition.

Perhaps this is the first time in a long while when you felt really good. Let me assure you, there is a fountain of youth. It isn't a drinking fountain, it's challenging physical training.

Now that you have gotten back to solid physical training, you want to "thrive" instead of just "survive". That means building on your investment and begin training at the next level.

Sustaining Activities

After three months on this program, you have probably found some activity that you enjoy more than the others. For some this will be weight training. For others it will be more aerobic such as running, swimming, or cycling.

It doesn't matter which is your favorite. It is your key to staying fit for life because you *enjoy the process* of training for some recreational activity that engages your body and your mind.

If you enjoy a competitive sport that can be the focus of your training, consider getting more involved in that activity on a regular basis.

When I say "sport" I mean an activity that will require you to maintain good muscularity and require you to keep your cardiovascular system in good condition. I'm thinking of such sports as foot racing, tennis, swimming, racquetball, cycling or something more extreme such as martial arts.

While golf is a pleasant pastime, it places virtually no demands on your body of the kind that will keep you in good physical condition. I'm aware that many pro golfers work out very hard. If you want to follow their example, fine. However, the physical demands of golfing are not enough to keep you in shape.

Your long-term commitment will be to *the process* of training. You are *living* the fitness lifestyle year in and year out. As the old Nike add said "there is no finish line"

Whatever your choice of activity, embrace it with gusto.

Options for future training

You have built a foundation for using power training as the core of your future fitness program.

I strongly suggest using training programs for powerlifting as the best way to continue to build your strength and fitness. Powerlifting training conditions the whole body and can work for anyone regardless of age. You don't have to compete, but you can do the training and get the fitness and strength benefits.

Having competed in powerlifting for 25 years while having a full professional and personal life, I learned a lot about building strength, staying healthy, and enjoying the opportunity to compete. I traveled all over the world in my work, had a family, and social life.

I believe that power training enabled me to have the energy, fitness, and resilience to enjoy a full and varied life.

Being strong as you age is amazingly important. This has not just been my personal experience (now at age 78) but also many that of many I trained and others I knew. That is why I'm convinced that being strong is essential to having a good quality of life after age 50.

For you, I offer training programs that you can use to build (and keep) your body it top condition. These progressively more challenging programs can be found on my website:

www.MidLifeHardBody.com

If you feel ready to take on powerlifting training, then I strongly suggest you obtain my book *Powerlifting Over 50* on Amazon.com.

You can also allow me to develop a custom training program for you by contacting me at Richard@MidLIfeHardBody.com

I assure you that if you are serious about your training, and want good value for your money, these are excellent options.

You can check out my web site at www.MidLifeHardBody.com

I hope you enjoyed the "first three months of the rest of your life". There is more good stuff awaiting you in the future.

Appendix A

Setting Up a Home Gym

Training at Home: A Popular Option

Having equipment for doing a workout available in your home is a great idea. Home gyms can be either your primary place to train, or an option to use occasionally. It is not an "either-or" situation.

In this chapter I'll walk you through the process of evaluating what *you* need for your unique situation.

Let's begin with a couple basic questions.

Will the home gym be your primary or secondary place to work out?

The first question to answer is whether you intend to use your home gym as your primary place to do your workouts, or as a backup when you can't get to the gym.

If it is your primary workout location, you will have to ensure that the equipment you buy will meet all your training needs, not just some of them.

You really must avoid any impulse purchases of equipment. At a gym if you get tired of using a certain piece of equipment, you walk away and go to something else. At home, if you bought it, you will be stepping over (or around) it constantly.

How much space do you have?

How much of your home do you intend to devote to hosting workout gear? The answer will be different for almost everyone.

The word "home gym" conjures up many different images. The options range from a few devices that hide in a closet between uses to a fully dedicated location with a complete assortment of weights and machines.

People who have a three-car garage or a detached building on their property will have different constraints than someone who lives on the 39th floor of an apartment building in Chicago.

Your first consideration will be how much space you intend to dedicate to your own fitness spa.

This calculation is specific to you and your circumstances.

For example, when I lived in a 5000-square foot house with a 3-car garage, I had a full set of barbells and kettlebells with a power cage set up in my garage. Even though this was not my primary workout location, I had all the gear to replicate a full gym workout.

Now I live in a townhouse and use a different strategy for hosting my home workout equipment. My kettlebells and sandbags lurk in closets and behind doors when not in use. My pull up bar hides behind a door when not in use.

In brief, figure out how you will use the space you have available for your own version of the "home gym"

Make a Plan: Address your training needs

Your goal in setting up a home gym is to get good value from your investment. Will your money be well spent, and will you be able to attain your fitness objectives?

First, your training will include both aerobics and weights. There are a lot of options for meeting these needs.

For aerobic training your basic options are:

- Train outside (run, swim, cycle, row, etc.)
- Do high repetition sets with light weights in your home gym
- Buy aerobic training equipment (treadmill, etc.)

For weight training your options range from:

- A few carefully selected dumbbells or kettlebells
- A single barbell with weight plates
- A home gym equipped with power racks, barbells, kettlebells and assistance equipment

In short, you have a lot of options and choices to make.

Whenever you consider purchasing a piece of equipment, your thought process should go like this:

- What _results_ do I expect from using this piece of equipment?
- How many different exercises or training routines can I do with this equipment?
- Will I quickly outgrow this equipment?
- How will this equipment fit into the space I have allocated for my home gym?

The bottom line is "does buying this make sense for _you?_"

Let's look at each of these questions in a little more detail.

Expected results: It is important that you are realistic about what the exercise value of a piece of equipment may be. What are *you* going to do with this device and how often? Do you have a plan for training on this equipment?

Specific answers to these questions will help you avoid a purchase you regret later.

It is important not to buy some device because you believe it will motivate you to train. The unfortunate situation is that when people assume they will get motivation from buying equipment, this they use the equipment one or two times.

If you are realistic about what you can accomplish with various pieces of gear, and how often you will *actually* use it, you reduce the chances that you buy something that soon becomes included in a yard sale.

Versatility: When thinking about buying a piece of equipment, you should consider how many different exercises you can do with any piece of gear.

Free weights are almost infinitely versatile. You can do hundreds of different movements with a free weight. You can do lifts standing, sitting, or reclining.

Weight machines on the other hand will generally allow for a few movements, and those will generally be done while sitting or lying.

Unless you lift the treadmill, the only exercise you can do with it is run.

Keeping pace with your Progress: Will you "outgrow" the equipment you buy? If so, how quickly will this happen? This is a critical question you need to ask any time you consider buying something.

As you get in better condition, you will be increasing the intensity of the exercise you do. With free weights you can put on more weight to make an existing move more demanding. You can also increase the weight you use on a weight machine.

Some specialized gadgets such as an abdominal roller are a good value because even a few reps are challenging. You are unlikely to outgrow this device.

Other pieces of equipment such as balance balls, elastic bands, and pull up bars are relatively inexpensive and will be useful in almost any fitness program. You will not outgrow them because they can be adapted to most any training intensity.

Logistics Issues: How difficult will it be to get this gear into your home? Will the vendor deliver it to the place you want to use it? Where will you store it when not in use? Does it require regular repair or maintenance?

These are the practical questions that must be answered when you consider buying equipment. Everyone will have different answers based on their situation. But, answer them carefully to avoid buying something you will regret later.

Getting value from home exercise equipment: Avoid the "Reverse BMW" paradox

Regardless of how much money you have, when you buy something you want to get value for your purchase.

If you are buying a car, you know that if you spend the money to get a BMW, it is going to give you top flight performance. If you buy a used Saturn with 200,000 miles on it, you won't get the same performance.

Oddly enough when I examine the equipment available for home fitness use, I find that the in *some* cases the exact opposite situation is true. The very expensive equipment gives far less value than expect for the price. I call this the" reverse BMW" paradox.

When I visit exercise equipment stores I notice that the sales floors have a lot of the equivalent of $10,000 toilet seats. These are big glitzy machines that promise to turn you into a fitness model in "20 minutes a day".

While the machines make it easier to do certain exercises, with few exceptions, they give vastly inferior results to free weights. But, over the past decades, people have become conditioned to think of machines as critical to fitness.

Given the public belief in exercise machines, commercials now abound showing men and women with god like appearance using the expensive toys implying that they got their "look" by "training 20 minutes a day three times a week" with this gizmo. The models looked great *before* they did the adds. Few ever trained on the equipment they are selling.

The hopeful and unwary can be persuaded by these fanciful demonstrations.

Bottom line: think long and hard before you buy any equipment, especially machines.

Aerobic Training Devices

As noted above, there are five types of aerobic training machines: treadmills, ellipticals, rowers, cycles and stair climbers.

Each of them gives a different type of workout, but basically their purpose is to get you in motion so that you elevate your heart rate for a period of time.

Each device involves moving your arms and legs differently so that you get some muscular conditioning from this action.

Treadmills

Before you embrace my opinions on treadmills, I should disclose that in the 50+ years I have been running 3-6 times a week, I have used a treadmill for my running workout exactly twice. Both times it was because of a snowstorm (Moscow, Russia and Frankfurt, Germany).

This experience does not exactly qualify me as an expert on treadmills. However, I have helped move them for friends, and can attest to their weight and bulk.

I find that people like treadmills because for them running outside is either uncomfortable, inconvenient, or unsafe.

If you strongly prefer treadmill training, then the main question you need to answer before buying one is whether you will use it enough to justify the purchase price.

Treadmills are expensive, and they can only be used for running and walking. They are basically one trick pony's.

You should ask yourself if you will outgrow what the treadmill can do. If you get into good condition, you may switch to running outside. You may want challenges the treadmill cannot provide. Again, issues to consider before putting your money down.

Lots of fitness machines, including treadmills, wind up in garage sales. In one way this is sad. Usually, the seller bought the device originally with high hopes. The fact that the machine is for sale often means that the owner gave up on their dream of being fit.

Other Aerobic Machines

This includes rowing machines, cycles, stair climbers, and elliptical trainers.

Your bottom line on purchasing any aerobic training device should be "will it give me what I want?" and "will I use it regularly?".

As you can see these machines have a big "footprint". They can take up some serious floor space. If you don't use the machine a lot, it's kind of like having a freeloading friend move into your house and take up a bunch of space with his crap.

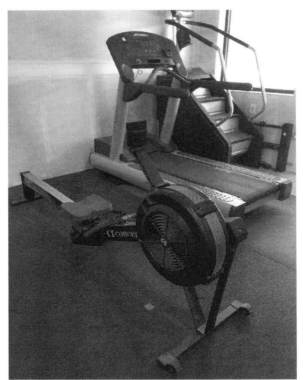

These devices are not cheap. A quality rower will cost several hundred dollars, and the same for the other gadgets. You can find cheap rowers for about $100, but you get what you pay for.

The same applies to exercise bicycles. Good ones cost a bunch, and cheesy ones don't give you much.

Bottom line: think long and hard before you buy a big piece of equipment. If you don't use it a lot, it is a bad investment.

Weight Training Equipment

When thinking about outfitting a home gym, there are basically two type of weight equipment you should start thinking with the least complicated solution.

If you have limited space, there is nothing that will give you more return on your investment than kettlebells. I have used kettlebells extensively for over 15 years, and when it comes to a great fitness tool that takes up almost no storage space, kettlebells are the undisputed champion.

The principal advantage kettlebells have over conventional dumbbells is that they can be used in a huge variety of exercises, some of which are movements unique to kettlebells.

Let's say that you live in an apartment in New York (or San Francisco). Floor space is at an absolute premium. You can get three kettlebells of different weights that fit under your bed when not in use. With these you can get both a great aerobic and a mind-blowing weight training workout.

To do these workouts you would only need the floor space required to stand up and extend your arms out in front of you.

If you have more space, but not a lot more, you can add kettlebells of different weights, or get pairs at the same weight.

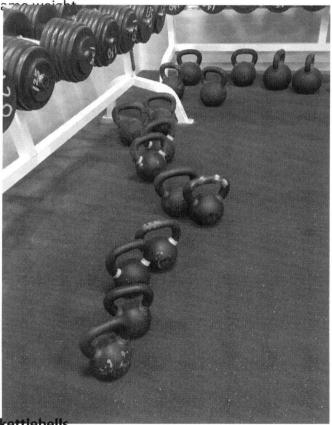

Purchasing quality kettlebells

If you buy a kettlebell there is a high probability that you will continue to use it for years. These delightfully sinister looking devices are simple in design, and there is a huge range of exercises you can do with them.

If you are outfitting a home gym, the kettlebell should be at or near the top of your list for a cost-effective fitness investment. They store easily in a small space, and never break down. Unless you toss it on the concrete, the bell should be just as good 100 years from now as it is today.

The kettlebell is basically a cannonball with a handle. Given the simplicity of the design, I have been amazed to find that some manufacturers can screw up even this simple design.

When you buy a kettlebell, you should check the dimensions of the handle. This is because some of the best kettlebell exercises require flipping the device overhead. If the dimensions of the handle are off, the bell will not rotate properly when you do the snatch or the clean, and you will get a very painful collision on your forearm.

The picture above shows the proper distance between the top of the handle (roughly 4 inches) and the body of the kettlebell. When you buy kettlebells make certain that you take this measurement.

Another design feature to consider is the finish on the handle. Many kettlebell exercises involve doing a high number of repetitions. If the finish does not allow the bell to rotate easily in your hand, you may wind up with painful blisters.

Like I said, it seems impossible to screw up such a simple design, but some manufacturers have.

IMHO there are three manufacturers that make outstanding kettlebells: Rogue, RKC, and Apollo. I would recommend them without the slightest hesitation. I own some from each manufacturer and use them all the time. Check my website www.MidLifeHardBody.com for recommendations on kettlebells and other home fitness equipment.

FYI: Kettlebells come in both pound sizes and kilograms.

If you are making your first purchase, I would recommend that you get three kb's of different sizes. You will be working out with them using one hand at a time.

If you are a man 5'7" and 160 pounds I would recommend getting 12Kg, 16Kg and 20Kg. If your store sells them in pounds: 25-35-45 pounds.

If you are a man taller than 5'7" and weigh more than 160 pounds, I would start with 16Kg, 20Kg and 24Kg (or 35-45-55 pounds).

Trust me, you will never outgrow these delightfully sinister conditioning tools.

Dumbbells

For the last decade or so, dumbbells have primarily been made only at fixed weights. In gyms you see a dumbbell rack with pairs of weights ranging from 5 lbs to well over 100 lbs.

If you are trying to set up your own home gym, fixed weight dumbbells are a problem because to make 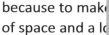 slates into a lot of space and a lo

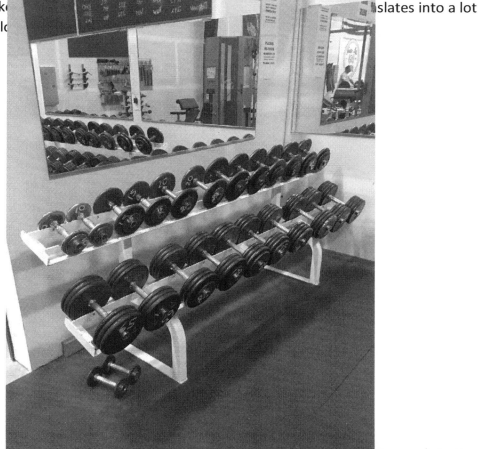

The picture shows a rack of dumbbell pairs that goes from 5 pounds to 85 pounds in 5-pound jumps. This is a lot of hardware!

IMHO the value of dumbbells in a home gym has been significantly diminished (or maybe even eliminated) by kettlebells.

The mainstay of weight training either at home or in a gym is going to be the barbell. At this point in time I usually recommend that people setting up a home gym don't bother to buy dumbbells unless they have: 1) a lot of space; and 2) plenty of money.

Weight Training Equipment

The primary piece of weight training equipment in a serious home gym is going to be a barbell. If you have the space for a 7-foot barbell and want to be able to do your primary weight training at home, that device will be your primary training tool.

In the recent past, the quality of home exercise weight lifting equipment has increased significantly. It is possible to get excellent value for a reasonable price.

This is good news for those who may be setting up home workout rooms.

Seven-foot-long bars, with associated plates, are available through a variety of outlets, including the intern̶e̶ _____ ods stores such as Dicks Sporting Good _____ e" barbells.

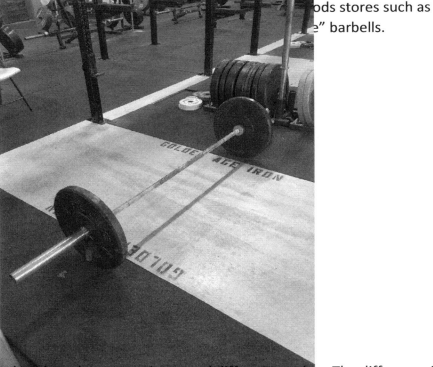

You should be aware that these bars come in several different grades. The difference is that some of them are built to the demanding specifications of competitive weight lifting. You need only get the bars that are good enough to use for a workout. That is the type you will find in most general-purpose gyms.

The picture on the left shows a 7' bar with rubberized "bumper" plates.

Metal plates are by far the cheaper option when compared to rubberized "bumper" plates. Rubberized _training_ plates for training are cheaper than those for competition.

The difference has to do with rigid specifications that have to be met for competition weight equipment.

As rubberized training plates become more popular, the price may continue to drop, so it is wise to compare prices before buying plates.

If you are setting up your home gym for the first time, you should be able to find a suitable bar and a set of metal plates for around $200. Rubberized plates are more expensive.

If you find you want to add weights later, individual plates are for sale from stores and on-line vendors.

Racks and Benches

One of the biggest positive changes in the home gym equipment area has been the significant improvement in the quality (and price) of racks and benches. The new gear is designed to allow for safe

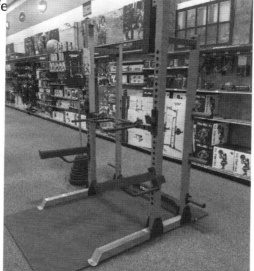

The rack is necessary to do any heavy lifting in the squat or the bench press. The new racks have adjustable safety bars that can be set to different heights, so you don't need a spotter to save you if you miss a lift.

Either of the racks shown above can be used for squatting or bench pressing. Both racks are relatively light weight. They should be adequate to handle weights up to 400 pounds. For heavier weights, the red colored rack is a heavy-duty multi-purpose rack.

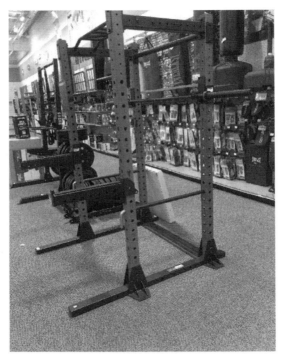

You need to select a bench that will enable you to train on the bench press as well as many other training lifts. The one pictured in the photo on the left is a multi-purpose bench that can be converted to four different incline settings.

You can also buy a simple flat bench that does not incline. It is mobile and can be moved in and out of the racks depending on what exercise you want to do.

It is not necessary to have a separate bench press bench. In the photo below, you can see how a mobile flat bench, like the one at the right, can be placed in a power cage for bench pressing.

You set the adjustable rack hooks to a position where you can take the bar for your bench press. Set the safety bars at a point just below where you touch your chest so that you can leave the bar on these bars if you can't complete the bench press

In the next photo you see a top of the line competition grade bench press bench.

Your principle concern is whether the bench will be sturdy and stable enough for your lifting. Some cheap benches are designed to support only light weight loads. Think about not only where you are starting, but how much weight you intend to be using in the next year.

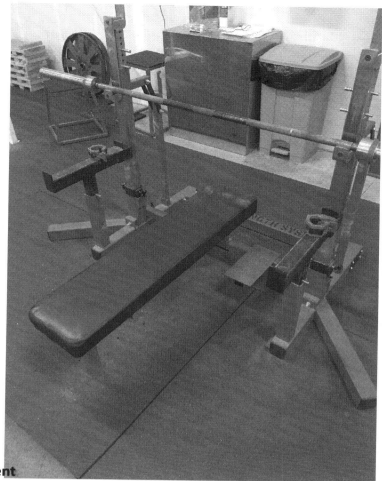

Other Equipment

You can invest in a few pieces of inexpensive equipment that will add a great deal to both the challenge and the versatility of your bodyweight workouts.

The first is a chinning bar that fits in a doorway. The second is a small wheel device that you use to do upper body strengthening.

Chin up/Pull up

The chin up or pull up is one of the greatest strength builders ever devised. It requires having a chinning bar and perhaps some assistance bands.

If you invest in a chinning bar for your home, you can do not only the chins and pullups, but other great exercises such as hanging leg raises.

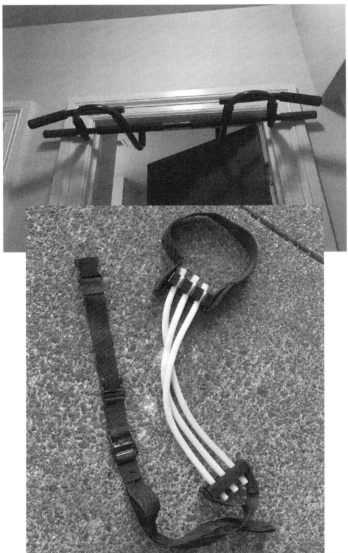

This picture shows a door mounted chinning bar that you can use at home. It attaches in the doorway by using a bracket that holds the bar in place against the molding. You put it up and take it down each time you use it.

You can find one of these bars by going to my web site www.MidLifeHardBody.com and going to the on-line store. They will be sent from Amazon, I have just made them easy for you to find.

Strength building begins when you can hold on to a chinning bar and have the grip strength to hold your bodyweight.

If you are just getting back into condition, you may need to use some assistance equipment to allow you to do chin ups and pullups.

IMHO the best device for this is an "chinning assistance band". As shown in the picture above, this is a nylon strap that can be looped over a chinning bar, a set of elastic bands to provide lift, and a stirrup in which to place one foot.

Depending on the strength of the elastic band, you can get anywhere from 20 to 50 extra pounds of assistance on your pullups.

Over time you will build up to doing sets of 20-30 at a time, and 100 or more in a week.

Eventually you want to be able to do many pullups (or chins) with minimal assistance. However, using assistance bands will help you progress far more rapidly than if you had to struggle doing only unassisted chins.

I also have an Amazon link in my on-line store to help you find these devices on my web site at www.MidLifeHardBody.com

Abdominal Wheel

This device allows you to build serious strength in all your core muscles as well as your arms and shoulders. It is a deceptively simple device, but regular use will give you phenomenal strength.

The abdominal wheel design is basically the one shown in the picture below. Different vendors offer different styles of the same basic design. They all do the same job.

The basic movement is straightforward. Begin kneeling on a floor or on a soft pad or folded towel so that your knees are comfortable. Grasp the wheel with both hands and place it on the floor in front of you.

Slowly roll the wheel out in front of you, keeping your arms relatively straight. Almost immediately you will notice that this movement puts a lot of stress on your arms, shoulders, and core. Beginners should be aware that this exercise can get difficult very quickly.

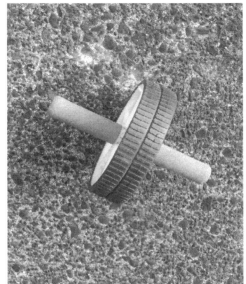

Only roll the wheel out in front of you as far as you can without feeling too much stress. You should think about building up gradually to the point where you can roll the wheel out in front of you so that your arms are fully extended over your head, and your chest touches the floor.

No matter whether you are a beginner or have done years of training, the "ab wheel" can give you a great workout.

You can buy one of these by visiting my site at www.MidLifeHardBody.com and going to the online store tab.

As you progress further in your training, there are many pieces of equipment that will give you a lot of exercise for your money.

Not normally used by beginners but used regularly by experienced lifters are elastic bands that have different tension strengths.

The idea behind bands is that they change the demands of a lift by altering the load you are lifting at different parts of the lift. Think of exercise bands as being giant rubber bands that you attach in different ways to bars to either increase or decrease the weight you are lifting.

Bands are a mainstay of power training around the world. The picture below shows the selection of bands available at the gym where I do most of my training.

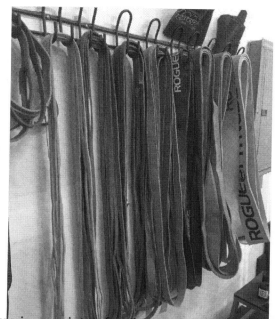

As you can see they come in a variety of resistance strengths. The ones on the left provide minimal resistance, while the thicker bands on the right provide some serious resistance.

Other Lifting "stuff" you may want at some point

There is a lot of fitness equipment for sale that I put in the category of "a solution in search of a problem". Much of it is sold to the unwary, and soon becomes filler in yard sales.

However, there are some miscellaneous items you may want to consider as your training becomes more advanced.

Wraps for the knees and wrists are regularly used by competitive lifters. In the early stages of your training career I do not advise that you use either as they reduce the load your body should be learning to carry on its own.

Knee and wrist wraps are for advanced lifters, and generally used only when lifting maximum weights, and in competition.

If you get into powerlifting, you will eventually use wrist wraps. If you lift in what is called "support gear", you will also use knee wraps.

Gymnastics chalk is a universally used grip enhancer. The only drawback is that if you are not careful it can make a mess in your training area.

If you begin doing strength sports, you will probably begin using chalk. Chalk is used in both competition and training in gymnastics, powerlifting, Olympic style weightlifting, and strongman completions.

Sand bags can be a useful addition to your home gym. They provide a change of the dynamics of lifting because the load is not as easily controlled in your hands.

Sand bags can be used to enhance both weight training and cardio training. They also provide a different type of resistance in that they are an odd shape for lifting, and the load shifts a little as you lift.

Sandbag workouts can help build coordination, balance, and endurance. I have used them off and on for a decade, and like them a lot.

From a logistical point of view, they are easily stored out of sight between workouts. You also only need one or two bags to have all the equipment you need.

My only caveat is that you may want to consider sand bags only after you have done enough weight training to get the most benefit out of them. In my view, they could be a useful addition to you home gym after you been training for at least three to six months.

Things you don't need: Lifting Belts and Gloves

There are pieces of equipment that are either useless or detrimental. Gloves and lifting belts head the list of "junk" you don't need.

Lifting belts are useful only when you are: 1) in top shape; and 2) doing a lift that is 90 or more of your 1 rep maximum.

When you are getting back in shape, lifting belts *retard* your progress. They take a portion of the load that your body should be getting in shape to handle. In short, the belt makes you *weaker* in your core, which is a place you really need to toughen up.

Some people will say, "I have a bad back". If you need a lifting belt to do any of the workouts in this book, or any beginners bodybuilding workout, you should be in physical therapy, not in training. Your doctor or physical therapist should clear you to do weight training before your start any workouts.

Wearing a belt when you are beginning training will weaken you. This is the opposite of what you want. As a rule, no one should wear a belt while they are doing conditioning training with light or modest weights.

Your goal should be to develop a "built in belt". A "core of steel" is your best protection against chronic pain and occasional injuries.

This is not just my opinion. I was first made aware of this viewpoint by the legendary Pavel of kettlebell fame. He wrote that one of the principles of Soviet/Russian training methods for strength athletes was to avoid using belts and consciously focus on building a "core of steel".

In the 25 years I spent as a competitive powerlifter, my own experience was that when I focused on building my own "built in belt", my back problems became nonexistent. Prior to that time, I had occasional issues with my back, but nothing serious.

The general rule that I used was that I never put on a lifting belt until I was at 90% of my one rep maximum for a given lift. This meant that my body was strong enough to lift big weights without the external support of a belt.

You may find it comforting to know that in my quarter century of competing, I was never seriously injured. Furthermore, I never had a minor injury that required me to miss more than a day or two of training.

So...build up your core (back, side and abdominals) so that you don't need a belt...except when lifting your one rep maximum.

Gloves

Gloves are another piece of equipment that you are better off without. Gloves will undermine your grip strength in a serious way. They prevent you from developing hands and fingers capable of holding significant weights.

As you progress in your conditioning, your grip will get stronger and stronger simply because you are handling weights.

The only valid reason I have ever encountered for using gloves is women who don't want to get callouses on their hands. Also, some women wanted to protect their fingernails. For the latter, I suggested that they use baseball batting gloves as those gloves cover the end of the finger.

For everyone else, either don't buy gloves in the first place, or toss them in the trash.

Home Training Facilities: The Long-Term View

If you opt to set up a home gym, you should think of it as something that will "grow and change" over the months and years.

You don't have to buy everything you think you might need right at first. My own experience has been that as you get more experienced at working out you will buy things that you actually use at home, and not buy things that you can use better at the gym.

You may also decide to get rid of some gear that you don't find useful or outgrow.

Keep an eye on the equipment available for home use as it changes over time, usually getting better or cheaper, or both.

Appendix B

Training while Traveling

When I first began regular business traveling in the 1970's, most people considered working out to be a form of mental illness.

Things are very different now. There are usually good gym's in almost any town. You will find people running on the street in the most remote locations on earth.

But, some issues will always be there, like traveling across time zones, and dealing with the disruption of your personal schedule. But, keeping up your training while traveling has become less of a problem over the past decades.

If your travel is a onetime event, such as a vacation trip, you can decide how much training you want to do before you depart. If you regularly travel, it is essential that you develop a plan to train at your destination to minimize the disruption to your program.

For over 30 years I regularly traveled from Seattle to the east coast of the US. One or two trips a month were part of my normal pattern. Through planning and a variety of trial and error learning, I learned how to train with minimal disruption.

There was a five-year period in my working career when I traveled internationally almost every month and tossed in a few domestic trips between the overseas jaunts. It was either learn how to train on the road or give in to the physical ravages of life on an expense account.

Travel by car presents some issues but going across several time zones is not one of them. You spend the day sitting in a car, but don't have to deal with the disruption to your body clock that you do when flying.

Success begins with a plan. If you have no plan, your plan is to fail!

Start by packing your workout clothes and any other training stuff you can't live without.

Next is planning what you will do when you are "there". For example, I regularly made 10-14-day trips to Russia and Ukraine (from Seattle). This meant planning at some serious workouts overseas.

Travel across many time zones introduces another wrinkle that you don't confront at home: jet lag.

The search for an antidote for jet lag has gone on for decades. Thus far, no Magic bullet.

I didn't develop a perfect solution but did come up with a method that minimized the disruption to my body clock.

First off, during the flight I was either working or sleeping. I found that if I slept for a large chunk of a long trip, the disruption to my bod was far less than if I stayed awake.

Second, drink lots of water. Airplanes cabins are like living in a food dryer. On a long trip you will become dehydrated. Drink at least one 8 oz cup of water for each hour you are in the plane. A bit more would be OK. Note that I said "water", not beer, wine, or soda. These dry you out.

Third, a mental trick that is easier said than done. Basically, tell yourself that whatever time it is at your destination is the time you will be "on". If you sit in your seat and wonder "will I be wasted when I get there?", you probably will.

Flying east is more disruptive than flying west. When you fly east (to Europe) you will be shortening your sleeping time. Suddenly you only have four hours of sleep instead of eight.

If you can manage it, when you arrive immediately start living on local time. Don't take a nap. Go to sleep at bed time at your destination. This can be grim at times.

If you have the luxury of taking a day or two before your trip to adjust to the time change, you can start living at home as if you were already at your destination.

Going west you chase the sun, and so you have the sensation of departing at one time, flying for a very long time, and arriving only a little bit after your left. For example, coming back from Moscow, we would leave about 2 PM, fly for nine hours and arrive in New York at 4 PM.

Chasing the sun is an easier adjustment, but you will still be fatigued.

But, back to what you do when you arrive at your destination.

When you arrive have a short workout. This will help you adjust to your new location.

If you are a runner, you should have minimal problems. In just about every city and town in the US (and Europe) running is a "normal" activity. Take a short leisurely jog (or treadmill session) and it will help you recover from the flight.

The same applies to weight training...just do enough to remind your body of the fun you have when you lift weights.

If you go to a gym, do several exercises with *light weights and high reps.* The purpose is to get moving again.

Stick in a few minutes of cardio on a treadmill or rower.

The whole purpose of this adaptation workout is to get rid of the body's "residue" from riding ten plus hours in a seat the size of a garbage can.

If you don't have access to a gym, do a few calisthenics in your hotel room. Pushups, deep squats, burpees, leg raises, etc. will do just fine.

Tell yourself that this is going to help you adapt to the time change. Your body may scream for a nap, but you are best off doing a light workout and going to bed on local time.

After you have been at your new location for a day or two, you can think about doing your regular workouts again.

Depending on your needs and desires, most big hotels these days have a "workout room". These are rarely adequate for power training, but they may have some useful equipment. Occasionally I found full barbell sets, and a good selection of dumbbells. Most often, the equipment was lame...but clearly better than nothing.

If you want to find a well-equipped gym, you should be able to find one on the internet either before you depart, or when you arrive.

The number of decent gyms around the planet has increased dramatically since I first began traveling. Now it is possible to find well equipped facilities almost anywhere.

This is especially true in the United States. Even the smallest town will usually have some type of weight training option. I even found a well-equipped power gym in a tiny town in one of the most remote parts of the US.

When you find a gym, the vast majority will allow you to pay for single workouts if you don't live in the area.

I have even managed to talk my way into high school weight rooms if there was no gym in town.

In the first few days after you arrive, the quality of your workout will probably not be what it would be if you were home. Your strength will be somewhat diminished, and your endurance not quite up to what it would be at home.

After 2-3 days, you may be able to do what would be a regular workout for you. Your bod will have adjusted to the time change, and you will have shaken off the effects of the flight.

Depending on the length of your stay, and your work commitments, you can train pretty much as if you were home.

If you don't have access to a good gym, keep up the bodyweight training in your hotel room. You will most likely be pleasantly surprised at how well this keeps your strength up.

One thing you should NOT do is use your travel as an excuse to pig out at meals and abandon any semblance of training. It is too easy to say, "coach never taught me how to live on an expense account", or "on vacation, anything goes".

The bottom line is to plan, and you can travel with minimal disruption to your training program. This is particularly true if you travel on a regular basis to the same locations.

Plan Ahead

You can use the internet to scout out potential workout venues in the area where you are traveling. This can make it a lot easier to keep up your training.

You should also plan for the weather condition where you will be visiting. If you go to a "winter" destination pack the right clothing for the location where you will workout.

Appendix C

Treating Routine Muscle Pain and Injury

Minor muscle injuries occur with some regularity. These are usually manifest as having "sore" muscles, having a very tender spot in your muscles or on a tendon, or having your range of motion limited by pain in certain positions.

The most common muscle injuries come from some type of overuse. They are often found as very sore or tender spots. These are called "trigger points" and are essentially knots and tangles of muscle tissue. They are very inflamed and will persist or expand if not treated. The main way to treat these is with ice therapy or with message therapy. This will be discussed later.

Minor tendon injuries are show up as a sore spot on the tendon. Again, this is an inflammation much like the trigger points in muscle tissue. These injuries will spawn more injuries if they are not treated.

There are several things you can do to limit the likelihood of getting these injuries, and some things you can do to treat them when they do happen.

Basic Injury Prevention Steps

Tip 1. Start slow and build up gradually.

When you begin an activity that stresses muscles you have not used in a while, it is ALWAYS best to begin training at a low intensity. In weight training, I always advise everyone to begin with light weights and relatively high repetitions so that you are conditioning the muscle for more demanding loads as you get in better condition.

You should NEVER do an exercise "to failure" or anywhere close to it during your first month of doing a new training movement. You are far better off "blowing off" a set of exercises, or a certain movement if you are fatigued or if you don't "feel right".

Training at low intensity while you are developing the resilience to do harder loads is not easy to do. The "social pressure" of keeping up with your gym friends or other people in the class is always there. You need to be tough about this and skip movements when you don't feel right. The only person who's going to get hurt is YOU...not the person you think is watching. You are not going to become a super human from the effort you put out in one work out. However, you CAN become injured and slow or stop your progress.

Let's assume for the moment that you have been training for some time and are well conditioned for one sport or activity. Assume for the moment that you are a dynamite tennis player, but you want to add some weight training. You need to follow the same gradual approach to building up your strength and resilience. Your body is well trained for one activity but needs to be introduced to the "new" conditioning gradually. Take it slow at first, and you will be amazed what you can accomplish.

I suggest the gradual build up approach whether the person training is age 50 or 20. It is more important for the 50-year-old because frankly, we take longer to heal from an injury, and are more likely to get discouraged and quit if we get injured. You can achieve mind blowing results, but these results come from training consistently over time, and staying away from the injury bug.

Tip 2. Warm up properly and stay warm during exercise.

Warming up is something that most people who exercise take casually. Often this leads to an unwanted muscle injury, and occasionally worse. You don't need to take a huge amount of time to warm up, but it is important to get your muscles ready to perform. Here are some simple steps you can take that will help you warm up properly.

Dress so that you are warm throughout the training session or event. Your muscles will respond better if you are warm, but not overheated. If needed, dress in layers so that you can shed clothing as your body warms up.

The purpose of a warm up is to get your blood flowing to all parts of your body and remove any stiffness in your muscles before taking starting to move quickly. For most people the best way to do this is to do some SLOW jogging for about 2-3 minutes' maximum.

It is not a good idea to "stretch" a cold muscle. You should be somewhat warm before attempting any stretching. Stretches during the warm up should not be intense, but rather should help you ease into more vigorous activity.

Take a few moments to *gently* move your arms through the range of motion you will be doing in your training. This will help loosen joints and muscles. The emphasis should be easy movement rather than any sort of stress.

Do some easy knee bends without any weight. Again, the idea is to get flexible and warm while putting out a minimal effort.

At this point you should be ready for any activity specific warm up that you regularly use. For example, if you are a swimmer, you should be ready for some easy laps. If you are a golfer, you should be ready for some practice swings.

If you train regularly, one thing that I have learned in the sport of powerlifting is that it is a good idea to "practice" your warm up with the same diligence that you practice your sport or activity.   In my case, the training session consists of lifting some *very heavy* weights. To be ready to do this I carefully practice a warm up routine that enables me to go from a cold start to being able to produce an all-out exertion. This warm up does not take much time…. but it does take a lot of focus.

Warming up will help reduce the muscle injuries that come from not being ready to exert. These are the most common type of muscle injury, but they typically disrupt your workout program for days or weeks at a time.

One final note on warming up; it is a good idea to keep warm during your training session. When your body is hot, the air will seem cold, and often this will lead to sub-optimal performance and occasionally muscle injury. Don't be afraid to take clothing off and then put it back on later if you feel a chill. Stay warm…. stay loose…

Tip 3. You are better off doing less than you are doing too much.

Earlier I briefly discussed the risks associated with training too hard when you first start to work out. Men seem to be unable to go easy when they are getting back into shape. The tendency to overwork is far more prevalent than the inclination to do too little.

Reality is that "over training" has the potential to do lots of damage to your body, and certainly disrupt any training program you may be on. Over the decades, I have competed in weight sports I have seen several people who performed well below their potential because they did far too much work and were either tired or suffering from one injury or another.

When you begin a comeback, or begin training for the first time, remember that the sky is the limit to what you *can* accomplish. The issue for you is training *smart* not training too hard. In In this case, being "smart" means that you clearly understand what you can reasonably accomplish in any given training session, and not go too far beyond that. There is a very fine line between doing something at your maximum capacity and getting hurt. Most of us have found where the line is through trial and error…. mostly error.

There is an old expression found in gyms around the world "no pain, no gain". I want to assure you that after 60+ years of competing in sports, the phrase should be "no pain, no suffering". I don't mean to imply that physical training is easy or does not take hard effort. However, there is a big difference between pushing yourself per a systematic training plan, and merely working so hard you hurt yourself.

At any stage of your training, if you don't feel like it is a good idea to do a given set, or play another round, *don't do it!!!!!* This is especially true when you are first starting out, or just getting back into shape. The idea that progress comes from relentlessly pushing yourself every workout or match is strictly for the people who never win anything. If you don't feel like pushing yourself on a given day…don't push.

To illustrate the point, I'll use the example of a friend of mine who is a very good competitive lifter. Unfortunately for him, he rarely heeds my advice about pulling back during a workout if you don't feel up to the challenge. During one particularly intense training session he was pulling heavy deadlifts, and after two reps was fully spent. But, his program said "do 3", so he pulled with all his might. Net result: he ruptured one Achilles tendon, and tore a hamstring muscle. He had two surgeries and took a year to recover.

This is an extreme case, but the point is that you must use your mind if you are really going to build your body.

Tip 4. Good nutrition is critical if you want to be free of pain.

This should be a no-brainer, but most people overlook the fact that a lot of the "aches and pains" we experience are the consequence of poor nutrition. Junk food and lots of sugar will give you inflammation and digestive problems, not to mention overloading your liver processing toxic waste.

If you are serious about ridding yourself of pain, and building a strong and healthy body, it is you intend to build the body of an elite athlete, then you need to eat like an elite athlete.

By this I don't mean to jump on the Michael Phelps 12,000 calories a day diet…but rather that you eat nutritious foods at a caloric level designed to get you to an optimal body weight for your size and muscularity.

Tip 5: First Aid for Minor Injuries

The basic idea is not to get hurt in the first place, but if you do get a minor injury during training, there are some easy first aid methods used by athletes all over the world.

Ice-heat-and Advil: This is a general prescription that is used by everyone from the National Football League to everyday trainees. When you get an injury, put and ice bag on it. Keep the ice on the injury for about 10 minutes and then put a hot pack on it for another 10 minutes.

The ice speeds the flow of blood to the area, the heat expands the veins and capillaries, so the blood can move more freely. Alternate the ice and the heat 2 or 3 times.

If you sustain a more serious injury (one that does not clear up by itself in a day or so), you should contact a Sports Medicine Doctor. The physicians that specialize in sports medicine will be the ones that can get you back training as quickly as possible.

Doctors in general practice will not have nearly as much experience with sports injuries and may not be able to give you the most effective treatment.

Over time you should develop a list of therapists that can help you with training related injuries. These would include message therapists, sports injury clinics, and sports nutritionists.

Obviously if you sustain a significant injury head for the Emergency Room.

Tip 6: Look for a couple non-obvious causes of your pain: shoes and bed

Over many decades I have talked with people who had problems such as "sore knees", "sore back", "sore hip", etc.

Very often the source of their problem turns out to be in one or both of the following places:

- Their shoes are worn down and it is causing bad body alignment when they walk or run
- Their mattress is worn and is not giving them good support during sleep.

If you have pain in your legs, back, and/or hips, one of the first places to look for a cause is your shoes. Way too many people continue to wear shoes that are worn down on the heel. Your training and street shoes should not show any signs of wear on the heel.

If heels are worn down it creates a mis-alignment every time you take a step. If you walk or run on shoes with worn heels, it will distort each stride. You get unwanted pressures on the knees, hips and back when this happens.

Bottom line: one of the worst places to try and save money is on shoes. By that I mean quality not quantity.

Another place that can be the cause of back pain, neck pain, shoulder pain, etc. is a worn mattress.

You spend about 1/3 of your life in bed, and it is the time when your body is doing it's best to repair and restore itself. It makes no sense to sleep on a mattress where your body is put in distorted positions that put pressure on the spine, legs, et.

Check your mattress to see if it gives you firm support. There should not be any depressions or lumps in it. If it needs replacing, do it soon.

Appendix D

Finding a Gym that works for you

If you are beginning the process of getting back in shape, working out at a gym can have several advantages, and some disadvantages.

The big advantage is a lot of weights, and some other equipment that you may be interested in using later.

The big disadvantage to most people just starting back is the fact that the gym seems like a "foreign country" where a lot of the locals may appear threatening.

Another disadvantage of a gym is that you may be given a lot of sales pressure to hire one of their staff (personal trainer) to help you.

Let's look at how you would do your personal cost/benefit calculation for joining a gym.

Potential Benefits

Lots of weights, lots of equipment.

In terms of things to lift, most gyms will have a big selection of dumbbells, barbells and often kettlebells. In addition, they will have a variety of weight machines.

Most gyms of any size will have treadmills, rowers, stair climbers, stationary bicycles, and other aerobic training machines.

Depending on the facility, they may also have a swimming pool, tennis courts, squash and racquetball courts, basketball gyms, yoga studios, and so on.

Almost all gyms will have a locker room where you can change clothes and shower as well as lock your valuables in a locker. Many will have a sauna and steam room.

In short, the big advantage that gyms have is lots of "toys" that you can play with and don't have to buy.

Potential Burdens

The principle burdens of gym membership are how much it will cost you each month to belong.

This will vary widely. Some gyms in my area charge as little as $10 per month. A more common amount is $30-60 depending on the size of the facility.

Private clubs may charge much more. It all depends on the facility and what they offer.

One risk of joining a gym is that many require a one-year contract for membership. That means you pay the membership fee regardless of whether you use the facility or not.

earlier, most people quit within a month of signing up. They still had to pay off their contract.

Some require a "membership fee" to join. This can range from a modest amount to a significant sum if you are joining an exclusive country club type facility.

Whatever the actual dollar amount You should consider the monthly out of pocket cost of joining a gym before committing.

Other Potential Burdens

When someone who is not a "gym rat" joins a new gym, they often have that "deer in the headlights" look for the first few weeks. This is because they are feeling very uncomfortable in the new surroundings.

Part of the discomfort is that everyone else appears to know what they are doing and may seem unfriendly.

Mostly this is an incorrect perception.

Most know how to find the equipment they use. They may be completely lost when it comes to using unfamiliar equipment.

For example, I once belonged to a club that in addition to world class weight rooms, had very nice tennis facilities. Even though I was a member of the club for five years, I still had only a vague idea of which end of the tennis racquet to hold.

As for being unfriendly, often that is because people doing serious weight training tend to be very focused on what they are doing. If you lift heavy weights you will get killed if you let your mind wander.

Another thing that can be intimidating when you are just getting back in shape is the presence of some people who really are in great condition. These people often appear intimidating just because they may be totally "buff".

With a few exceptions, these people are the ones who will be most willing to help you or share what they know. In the past 60+ years of training in gyms, I have found that those who are the most fit are generally the most open to helping others.

There are a few exceptions. Hopefully, you won't encounter them.

In short, don't let your perception of the "social atmosphere" of a gym keep you away if it looks like it would be a good place for you to train. The locals will tend to warm up the more often they see you working out.

If you feel like you "don't belong" in a gym that is new to you, remember that everyone there probably felt that way when they started. After you have been there a few times, it will gradually feel more like "your place".

Logistics Issues

Before you sign up with a gym, you need to look at practical logistics issues that could have a big impact on how regularly you use the facility.

Is it open when you want to train? How crowded will it be at the times you want to work out? How far do you have to travel to get there? Is the parking adequate at the times you want to use it? Do they have onsite day care if you need that?

It is important to think about these things before you commit to a certain place, because they can become a huge factor if they create problems for you later.

Some Bad Reasons for Joining a Gym

If you believe that by making the commitment to join a gym, and pay the monthly bill, you will motivate yourself to work out regularly, forget it. It doesn't work that way.

Joining a gym will motivate you one or two times, and after that, it will be easy to blow off. Remember, 90% of the people who join a gym will quit within a month.

Your motivation to train and get back into good condition must come *before* you join the gym.

Another bad reason for joining a gym is that someone who promises to work out with you trains there.

Sorry, but "workout partners" are inherently unreliable. Their schedule and priorities may not align with yours. They may be less committed than you. They may have a completely different goals than yours for why they want to work out.

There are any number of reasons why it is unwise to select a gym because you believe another person will train there with you.

The exception to this would be if they were part of your family. I know of several husband-wife training pairs as well as father-son, mother-daughter, etc.

In my 60+ years of training I have yet to have a "workout partner" who showed up on a consistent basis. Roughly 99% of the time I had no workout partner at all.

It is a poor idea to make your working out in any way dependent on another person who may not have your commitment.

Summary: Your personal "cost/benefit" analysis

When you consider all the factors that go in to deciding to join a gym, you can do your own informal cost benefit analysis of any given facility.

The costs are straightforward: time, money, and effort.

The benefits are whether *after careful consideration* believe that you will use the gym *at least a dozen times a month.*

The costs will always be there. You need to assure yourself that every month you will visit the gym at least a dozen times. If not, why not?

These are questions that only you can answer.

Appendix E

Bodyweight Exercises

Bodyweight exercises or "calisthenics" are an underappreciated form of conditioning. If you are getting back into shape after age 50, you can get great benefits from doing bodyweight exercises.

It is useful to think of bodyweight exercises as *complementary* to lifting weights. Both are resistance training, but they will condition your body in different ways.

Bodyweight training will promote developing *athletic strength and flexibility*. That is, the ability to do complex movements that require strength, coordination, and muscular endurance.

Think for a moment about the nearly astonishing strength and conditioning gymnasts and wrestlers have. You will find almost no one who lifts weights exclusively who has either the strength or athleticism to do even elementary routines on the still rings, pommel horse, or parallel bars.

If you are over 50 you can regain mind blowing strength by practicing bodyweight movements regularly.

I include bodyweight movements in this book for two reasons. First, as an *option* to be used as a part of your regular training, and second as a workout you can do if you can't do your regular training.

Program design

The exercises listed below are intended to *re-introduce* you to bodyweight training. You have probably done most (or all) of these exercises at some time in your life. However, it is unlikely that you did them consistently.

Each of these exercises place different demands on the entire body. There is no *isolation* movement. While some muscle groups may carry most of the load, each of these movements is a *whole-body* exercise.

The idea is to gradually increase your capacity to do a greater total number of reps in each exercise. Rather than try to max out the number of reps you do in one set, your aim is to build up the _total number of reps you do each workout, and the total volume of work you do in a week._

1. The "Jack Knife"

This is a combination warm up and conditioning movement. You will get good muscle activation for the entire body. It will also help you condition some weak links you may have.

The jack knife works all of your core (front and back) as well as your arms and shoulders.

Begin on the floor with your hands placed slightly wider than shoulder width. This is the starting "push up" position. You will have your toes turned under and feet slightly wider than shoulder width.

The first move is to push your trunk upward while keeping your hips on the floor. At this point, raise your hips up and pushing with your arms straight, raise your butt into the air. You will be on your hands and your toes with your tail end in the air.

This may not be the coolest look in the gym, but if you do this regularly you will get to be cool all the rest of the day.

Lower your hips until they are almost touching the floor. Get a good stretch in your lower back and a good extension in your abs.

Start out and see how you feel doing 5-10 reps for 2-3 sets. It may take a while, but keep adding reps until you can do *50 non-stop reps.*

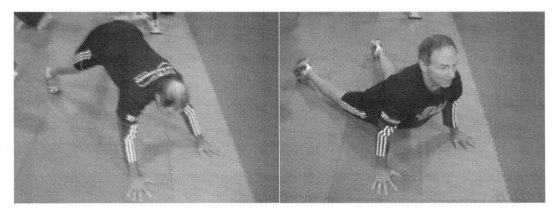

When you first start doing this movement, you will probably find that it is hard to do more than a few reps before some part of your bod is heavily taxed. As you train more, that weakness will go away, and you will have balanced strength.

Work up slowly, and you will find that gradually the weak links in your power chain have been brought up to where the others are.

2. Squat

There is no exercise that is more critical....or more disliked...than the squat. The squat will give you conditioning that nothing else can match or even approach.

In the free-standing squat, the intention is to lower yourself into a position where your hips are well below your knees.

For some of you at the beginning of this program, doing a deep squat will be impossible. Years of not getting in to a squat position will have left weak muscles stiff joints.

If this is the case, you should begin training by doing *partial* squats. That is, lowering your hips to a point where you can stand back up without assistance. Your goal is to *gradually* go deeper until you can do a full squat.

If necessary, start by holding on to a stable object so that you don't get stuck in a low position. You should gradually wean yourself from using any external support.

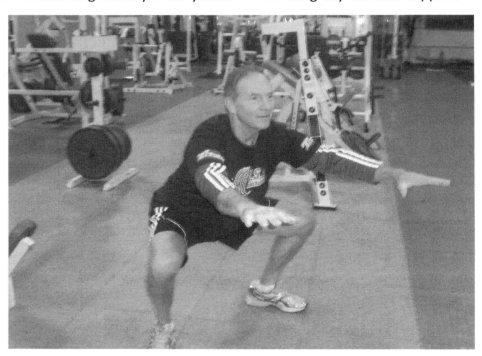

Begin standing upright with your feet a slightly wider than shoulder width. Your head should be erect throughout the movement. Keep your back flat, never rounded. Your arms can be crossed in front of you or hang down at your sides...your choice.

The proper way to squat is to descend by pushing your butt back as if you were going to sit in a chair. Do NOT bend your knees forward. *Lower your hips* while keeping your shins as vertical as possible. Push your knees slightly outward as you descend.

You should never allow your knees to bend forward so that they are out ahead of your toes. That puts a dangerous strain on your tendons and knee joints.

Your weight should be focused on the *inside half* of each foot. You should feel contact with the floor in the ball of your foot. Use the outside half of your foot for balance as needed.

To reach the bottom of the squat, you can use your hip flexor muscles to pull you into a low position. Initially, you can allow gravity to do the work, but eventually you want to have full muscular control throughout the lift.

When you reach the bottom of the squat, you begin the return to the starting position by making your chest lead the way as you stand up. There is a tendency for inexperienced trainees to begin coming out of the bottom of a squat by pushing they butt up in the air. Work on coming out of the bottom chest up....not butt up.

If you do the squat at a slow pace, you can release your breath when you return to a standing position. If you squat at rapid tempo, you may do a few squats before releasing your breath and inhaling again. Breathe at a pace that works for you.

Depending on your conditioning you may be able to do a few squats, or more than a few. You should begin with what is manageable, and gradually work up until you can do at least 30 nonstop reps. But...take your time getting there.

3. Pushup

The pushup is one of the most widely practiced conditioning movements of all time. Done regularly you will be amazed at what it will do for you.

Start on your hands and knees. Place your hands slightly wider than shoulder width on the floor. If you are strong enough, straighten your legs and balance on your toes. Feet should be roughly shoulder width apart.

Place a baseball sized object (about 2.5 inches) just below where your chest will be at the lowest part of the push up. This is what you will touch before you push back to the starting position.

The starting position is with arms fully extended, back straight, and legs straight. Take a deep breath and lower your chest to the floor. Keep your elbows in tight to your sides as you go down.

When your chest touches the ball, push yourself back to the starting position.

Depending on your conditioning at the start, do 3-5 sets of 5-10 reps. Take a short rest between sets.

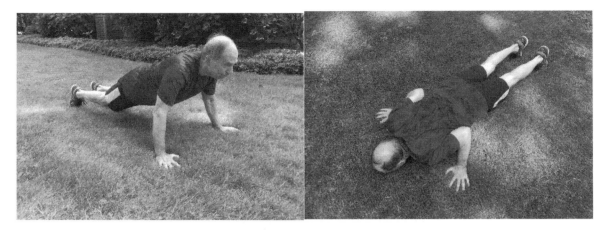

Initially you may do a total of between 25 and 50 reps for the session. When you feel up to it, add more sets to increase the total number of reps you are doing. Your goal should be to gradually increase the number of reps you do each session until you are doing a total of 50-100 reps each workout.

Initially you should not worry about the maximum number of reps you can do without a break. Work on building up the total volume of reps you do in a workout. This will allow you to make steady progress.

After a month of training, you may want to see how many pushups you can do in one set. But, don't start doing this every workout. It is not productive go for your limit more often than every two weeks.

4. Scorpion

This exercise will strengthen your lower back and help you develop more flexibility in your legs and hips.

Lie face down on the floor. Reach back with your right hand and touch the bottom of your left foot. To do this, you will bend your left knee so that your left foot is up against your butt.

Reaching back for your opposite foot will flex your lower back, and other muscles in your core.

You will alternate right hand to left foot and left hand to right foot until you have done a total of 10 reps on each side. Do 3 sets of this.

As you become more used to the movement, you should raise your chest off the floor as you reach back with either arm. This will make the exercise more intense, but also more beneficial.

Begin doing 2-3 sets of 10 and gradually work up to sets of 20-25.

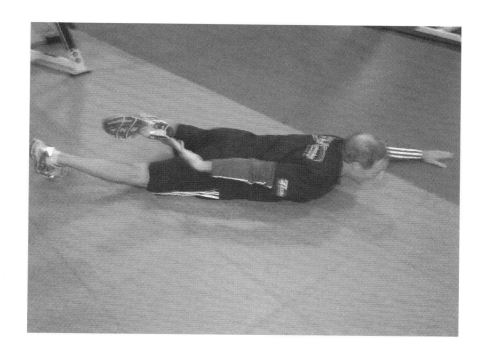

5. Back Bridge

This exercise is designed to strengthen your core and spinal support muscles. It will also work your neck and upper back.

Begin by lying on the floor with your feet pulled up near your rear end and your knees pointing at the ceiling.

Raise your hips off the floor until there is a straight line between your knees and your chin.

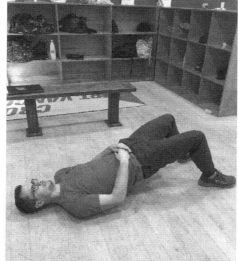

Initially you can put your hands on the floor if you need help raising your hips. As you become more proficient, you should keep your hands folded on your abdomen.

Begin doing 5-10 reps for 2-3 sets. Work up to the point where you can do 25 reps in a set.

6. Plank

The plank will give you a powerful core, particularly in the abdominal area.

Begin by lying on the floor propped up on your elbows. You should have a timer available that you can see easily.

The plank position will be where your weight is supported on your forearms and toes. Your back will be flat, legs straight, and you will be looking at the floor directly below your face.

Raise yourself into the plank position and hold your body rigid. You will be holding this static position for a specific time.

Initially, you will be holding the plank position for 10-15 seconds. When that becomes relatively easy, add 5-10 seconds.

When you have held the plank for your selected time, relax and allow your body to rest on the floor.

You should do at least 3 plank holds of 10-15 seconds each.

Gradually increase the time you hold each plank. Eventually you want to be able to hold each plank for 60-90 seconds.

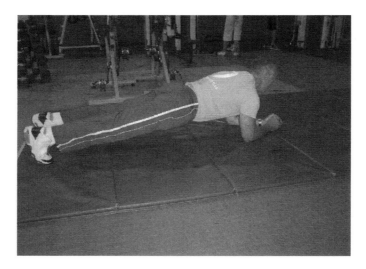

7. Leg Raise

Leg raises done while lying on the floor will give your core another challenge.

Lie on the floor on your back. When you first start doing this exercise, place your hands under your butt. As you get stronger, you can place your hands behind your head.

Take a deep breath and hold it. Keep your legs straight, and slowly raise them up until they are at a 45-degree angle with the floor. When you have reached this position, slowly exhale, and gradually lower your legs back to the floor.

Keeping a slow tempo is important in this exercise. It should take about 3 seconds for you to raise the legs to 45 degrees, and about 2 seconds to lower them back to the floor.

When you start doing this exercise, you should try to do 5-10 reps without stopping to rest. Gradually build up your strength until you can do 15-20 reps without a break.

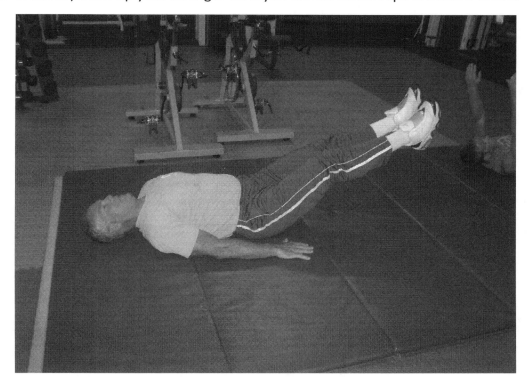

Bonus: Bodyweight Movements with Inexpensive Gear

You can invest in a few pieces of inexpensive equipment that will add a great deal to both the challenge and the versatility of your bodyweight workouts.

The first is a chinning bar that fits in a doorway. The second is a small wheel device that you use to do upper body strengthening.

8. Chin up/Pull up

This exercise is one of the greatest strength builders ever devised. It requires having a chinning bar and perhaps some assistance bands.

If you invest in a chinning bar for your home, you can do not only the chins and pullups, but other great exercises such as hanging leg raises.

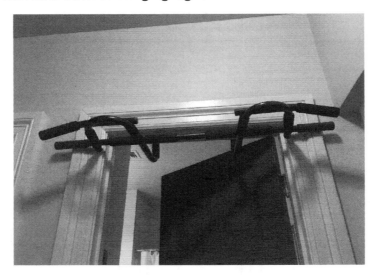

This picture shows a door mounted chinning bar that you can use at home. It attaches in the doorway by using a bracket that holds the bar in place against the molding. You put it up and take it down each time you use it.

You can find one of these bars by going to my web site www.MidLifeHardBody.com and going to the on-line store. They will be sent from Amazon, I have just made them easy for you to find.

If you train in a gym, one or more chinning bars will be available.

For people just getting back into shape, strict chinning and pullups can be quite difficult.

Strength building begins when you can hold on to a chinning bar and have the grip strength to hold your bodyweight.

The starting point for anyone getting back into shape is developing the strength to "hang" from a chinning bar gripping with both hands.

When you grasp the chinning bar you should tighten your entire body. You will not "hang" from the bar only using hand strength. You will *recruit* strength from all over your body. When you grip the bar, you should consciously tense every muscle in your body.

The effect of recruiting muscles to help hold your weight will be twofold: 1) your grip will be stronger; and 2) you will work a lot of muscles in your body that you might have thought would not be involved in pullups.

The first phase of training on the chinning bar will be to develop the ability to hold your bodyweight for up to a minute.

Like the plank exercise, you will develop strength by hanging from the bar for a few seconds and gradually increase the time you can hang on.

There are multiple options for gripping the bar. First the palms can face in (pullup) or palms can be facing away (chin).

You can select different widths to grip the bar. The narrowest is where your hands touch each other. Then move out to shoulder width. When the palms face away, a wider than shoulder width grip is popular.

Each grip variation works your body in a slightly different way. You should practice many different grip variations to develop (and maintain) good all-around strength.

The first hanging exercise is done with your hands roughly shoulder width apart, and palms facing in.

If possible, stand on a bench or something else that allows you to set your grip without supporting any weight. When you have placed your hands in the proper position, and are ready to hold your own weight, carefully step off the bench so that your hands have a few moments to adjust to holding your weight.

The next phase will be where you use some assistance equipment to allow you to do several repetitions of both chin ups and pullups that you could not do without help.

For this reason, I suggest that you begin by using some assistance equipment that will allow you to do multiple repetitions.

There are several readily available assistance devices. The most common is what is called an "exercise band". This is basically a big elastic band that you can loop over the chinning bar, and then place your foot in the bottom loop.

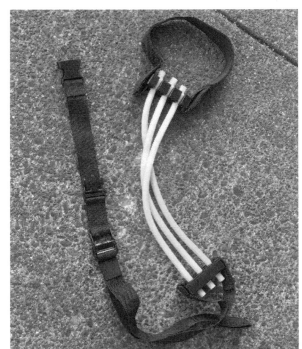

Depending on the strength of the elastic band, you can get anywhere from 20 to 50 extra pounds of assistance on your pullups.

I would recommend that you begin with a band that is strong enough to help you to do a five-rep set in both the chin up and the pullup.

When you can do five reps, then work until you can do at least ten reps before going to a lighter band.

Over time you will build up to doing sets of 20-30 at a time, and 100 or more in a week.

Eventually you want to be able to do many pullups (or chins) with minimal assistance. However, using assistance bands will help you progress far more rapidly than if you had to struggle doing only unassisted chins.

I also have an Amazon link in my on-line store to help you find these devices on my web site at www.MidLifeHardBody.com

Abdominal Wheel

This device allows you to build serious strength in all your core muscles as well as your arms and shoulders. It is a deceptively simple device, but regular use will give you phenomenal strength.

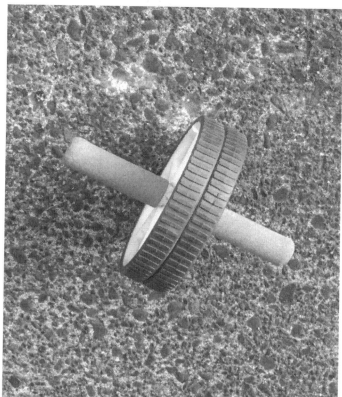

The basic movement is straightforward. Begin kneeling on a floor or on a soft pad or folded towel so that your knees are comfortable. Grasp the wheel with both hands and place it on the floor in front of you.

Slowly roll the wheel out in front of you, keeping your arms relatively straight. Almost immediately you will notice that this movement puts a lot of stress on your arms, shoulders, and core. Beginners should be aware that this exercise can get difficult very quickly.

Only roll the wheel out in front of you as far as you can without feeling too much stress. You should think about building up gradually to the point where you can roll the wheel out in front of you so that your arms are fully extended over your head, and your chest touches the floor.

Be patient. It may take many months to get to the point where you can do the full extension. As you build up your strength you will find that you can extend the wheel further out in front of you and have it under full control.

You can buy one of these by visiting my site at www.MidLifeHardBody.com and going to the online store tab.

Printed in Great Britain
by Amazon